SECTION 3 PRACTICAL PROCEDURES

SECTION 4 DRUG PRESCRIBING

SECTION 5 MANAGEMENT OF COMMON CONDITIONS

Symbols used in the text

 Important points

 Additional notes

CHURCHILL'S

House Physician's Survival Guide

For Churchill Livingstone:

Publisher Laurence Hunter
Project Editor Jim Killgore
Editor Therese Duriez
Production Nancy Arnott
Design Direction Erik Bigland
Sales Promotion Executive Marion Pollock

CHURCHILL'S

House Physician's Survival Guide

ROGER A. FISKEN MA DPHIL MD MRCP
Consultant Physician
Friarage Hospital
Northallerton, North Yorkshire, UK

Churchill Livingstone
EDINBURGH LONDON MADRID MELBOURNE NEW YORK AND TOKYO 1994

CHURCHILL LIVINGSTONE
Medical Division of Longman Group UK Limited

Distributed in the United States of America by
Churchill Livingstone Inc., 650 Avenue of the Americas,
New York, N.Y. 10011, and by associated companies,
branches and representatives throughout the world.

First published 1994

ISBN 0-443-04895-9

British Library Cataloguing in Publication Data
A catalogue record for this book is available from the British Library.

Library of Congress Cataloging in Publication Data
A catalogue record for this book is available from the Library of Congress.

The publisher's policy is to use **paper manufactured from sustainable forests**

Produced by Longman Singapore Publishers Pte Ltd
Printed in Singapore

PREFACE

This book is intended to supply the newly qualified house physician with up-to-date, practical advice about the many different aspects of the job which will be unfamiliar in the beginning. It is based on three principles which, in my experience, are given too little attention in most medical textbooks.

- Patients do not present to doctors with a diagnosis but with symptoms or, very often, diffuse problems for which there are several potential causes. Section 2 is, therefore, devoted to a wide variety of problems as they present in real life.
- Common things occur commonly. There is little point in knowing that breathlessness may be caused by bleomycin toxicity if you forget to consider asthma or left ventricular failure. The difference between the experienced doctor and the novice is, very often, that the senior person gives more weight to the most common potential causes of a problem and orders priorities accordingly.
- There may be situations in which it is as important (or more important) to treat than to perform a detailed clerking: the patient with severe cardiac chest pain needs venous access, pain relief, oxygen, thrombolysis and transfer to the coronary care unit at the earliest possible opportunity. Once he is stable on the unit, you can go on to ask about his employment history, previous fractures, etc. For some emergencies it is even necessary to have a 'mantra' in your head that you can recite as you run to the ward; in this way you can be more confident of remembering what to do and doing it in the right order.

The information in this book is as up-to-date as I can make it, but things change rapidly and if you are in doubt about something in the book, ask a more senior colleague or consult a recent reference source.

1994 R.A.F.

ACKNOWLEDGEMENTS

It is a pleasure to acknowledge the help and advice of many colleagues who have offered comments on this book. I am particularly grateful to Mr. John Taylor, sometime senior registrar in surgery at the Royal Liverpool Hospital, who made a major contribution to the chapter on intravenous fluids. Mrs. Pam Cross and Miss Claire Bickerton deserve warm thanks for their efforts in the typing of the manuscript. Finally, I must say especial thanks to my wife, Jenny, for her unstinting support while I was writing the book.

1994 R.A.F.

ABBREVIATIONS

A & E	accident and emergency
ABG	arterial blood gases
ACE	angiotensin converting enzyme
ACTH	adrenocorticotrophic hormone
ADH	antidiuretic hormone
AF	atrial fibrillation
AIDS	acquired immunodeficiency syndrome
ALL	acute lymphoblastic leukaemia
AML	acuyte myeloid leukaemia
ANF	antinuclear factor
APTT	activated partial thromboplastin time
ARDS	adult respiratory distress syndrome
ASD	atrial septal defect
ASO	antistreptolysin O
AST	aspartate transaminase
ATN	acute tubular necrosis
AXR	abdominal X-ray
BBB	bundle branch block
BD	bis diurnale (twice a day)
BMT	bone marrow transplant
BNF	British National Formulary
BTS	blood transfusion service
BP	blood pressure
CABG	coronary artery bypass graft
CAH	chronic active hepatitis
CAPD	chronic ambulatory peritoneal dialysis
CCF	congestive cardiac failure
CCU	coronary care unit
CLL	chronic lymphatic leukaemia
CML	chronic myeloid leukaemia
CMV	cytomegalovirus
CNS	central nervous system
COLD	chronic obstructive lung disease
COP	colloid osmotic pressure
CSF	cerebrospinal fluid
CSU	catheter specimen of urine
CT	computerized tomography
CVA	cerebrovascular accident
CVP	central venous pressure
CVS	cardiovascular system
CXR	chest X-ray
DIC	disseminated intravascular coagulation
DIP	distal interphalangeal
DM	diabetes mellitus
DVT	deep venous thrombosis
EBV	Epstein–Barr virus
ECF	extracellular fluid
ECG	electrocardiogram

EEG	electroencephalogram
ELISA	enzyme-linked immunosorbent assay
EMG	electromyography
ERCP	endoscopic retrograde cholangiopancreatography
ESR	erythrocyte sedimentation rate
FBC	full blood count
FEV1	forced expiratory volume in 1 sec
FFP	fresh frozen plasma
FSH	follicle stimulating hormone
FVC	forced vital capacity
GABA	gamma-aminobutyric acid
GFR	glomerular filtration rate
GGTP	gamma glutamyl transpeptidase
GH	growth hormone
GI	gastrointestinal
GIT	gastrointestinal tract
GKI	glucose/potassium/insulin
GN	glomerulonephritis
GVH	graft versus host disease
HBV	hepatitis B virus
HIV	human immunodeficiency virus
HLA	human leucocyte antigen
HSV	herpes simplex virus
IBD	inflammatory bowel disease
ICF	intracellular fluid
ICP	intracranial pressure
IHD	ischaemic heart disease
IM	infectious mononucleosis
IMHP	intramuscular high potency
INR	international normalized ratio
ISQ	idem status quo (i.e. unchanged)
ITP	idiopathic thrombocytopenic purpura
IVC	inferior vena cava
IVHP	intravenous high potency
IVU	intravenous urography
JVP	jugular venous pressure
KCCT	kaolin cephalin clotting time
LA	left atrium
LBBB	left bundle branch block
LFTs	liver function tests
LH	luteinizing hormone
LIF	left iliac fossa
LV	left ventricle
LVF	left ventricular failure
MCHC	mean corpuscular haemoglobin concentration
MCV	mean corpuscular volume
MEN	multiple endocrine neoplasia
MI	myocardial infarction
MIBG	meta-iodo benzyl guanidine

NSAID	non-steroidal anti-inflammatory drugs
OGTT	oral glucose tolerance test
OM	olim mane (once daily in the morning)
PA	pulmonary artery, pernicious anaemia
PCV	packed cell volume
PDA	patent ductus arteriosus
PEEP	positive end-expiratory pressure
PEFR	peak expiratory flow rate
PFTs	pulmonary function tests
PIP	proximal interphalangeal
PE	pulmonary embolism
PR	per rectum
PRN	pro re nata (as required)
PRV	polycythaemia rubra vera
PT	prothrombin time
PTC	percutaneous transhepatic cholangiogram
PTH	parathyroid hormone
PTT	partial thromboplastin time
PUO	pyrexia of unknown origin
QDS	quater diurnale summensum (four times a day)
RA	rheumatoid arthritis
RAST	radio-allergosorbent test
RBBB	right bundle branch block
RCC	red cell count
RIF	right iliac fossa
RVF	right ventricular failure
SLE	systemic lupus erythematosus
ST	sinus tachycardia
SVC	superior vena cava
SVT	supraventricular tachycardia
TB	tuberculosis
TBG	thyroid binding globulin
TDS	ter diurnale summensum (three times a day)
TIA	transient ischaemic attack
TIBC	total iron-binding capacity
TIP	terminal interphalangeal
TPN	total parenteral nutrition
TRH	thyrotrophin-releasing hormone
TSH	thyroid stimulating hormone
U&E	urea and electrolytes
URTI	upper respiratory tract infection
US	ultrasound
UTI	urinary tract infection
VF	ventricular fibrillation
VSD	ventricular septal defect
VT	ventricular tachycardia
VWF	von Willebrand factor
WBC	white blood count
WPW	Wolff–Parkinson–White

X BIOCHEMICAL VALUES

Venous blood: adult reference values

Analyte	Reference values	
Acid phosphatase (unstable enzyme)	0.1–0.4 i.u./l	
Alanine aminotransferase (ALT) (glutamin-pyruvic transaminase (GPT))	10–40 i.u./l	
Alkaline phosphatase	40–100 i.u./l	
Amylase	50–300 i.u./l	
α_1-Antitrypsin	2–4g/l	
Ascorbic acid — serum	23–57 μmol/l	0.4–1.0 mg/dl
— leucocytes	1420–2270 μmol/l	25–40 mg/dl
Aspartate aminotransferase (AST) (glutamic-oxaloacetic transaminase(GOT))	10–35 i.u./l	
Bilirubin (total)	2–17 μmol/l	
Caeruloplasmin	1–2.7 μmol/l	
Calcium (total)	2.12–2.62 mmol/l	
Carbon dioxide (total)	24–30 mmol/l	
Chloride	95–105 mmol/l	
Cholesterol (fasting)	3.6–6.7 mmol/l	
Copper	11–24 μmoi/i	
Creatinine	55–150 μmol/l	
Creatinine clearance	90–130 ml/min	
Creatine kinase (CK) — males	30–200 i.u./l	
— females	30–150 i.u./l	
Ethanol — marked intoxication	65–87 mmol/l	
— coma	> 109 mmol/l	
Ferritin — males	6–186 μg/ml	
— females	3–162 μg/ml	
α Fetoprotein	2–6 units/ml	
γ-Glutamyl transferase (γ-GT) — males	10–55 i.u./l	
— females	5–35 i.u./l	
Glucose (fasting)	3.9–5.8 mmol/l	
Immunoglobulins (Ig): IgA	0.5–4.0 g/l (40–300 i.u./l)	
IgG	5.0–13.0 g/l (60–160 i.u./l)	
IgM — males	0.3–2.2g/l (40–270 i.u./l)	
— female	0.4–2.5 gl (50–300 i.u./l)	
Iron — males	14–32 μmol/l	
— female	10–28 μmol/l	
Iron binding capacity (total)	45–72 μmol/l	
Iron binding capacity (saturation)	14–47%	
Lactate	0.4–1.4 mmol/l	
Lactate dehydrogenase (LDH)	100–300 i.u./l	
Lead	0.5–1.9 μmol/l	
Magnesium	0.75–1.0 mmol/l	
5' Nucleotidase	1–11 i.u./l	
Osmolality	285–295 mOsm/kg	
Phosphatase see acid and alkaline		
Phosphate	0.8–1.4 mmol/l	
Potassium	3.3–4.7mmol/l	
Protein — total	62–82 g/l	
— albumin	36–47 g/l	
— globulins	24–37g/l	
— electrophoresis (% of total)		
albumin 52–68		
globulin α_1 4.2–7.2		
α_2 6.8–12		
β 9.3–15		
γ 13–23		
Sodium	133–144 mmol/l	
Triglyceride (fasting)	0.6–1.7 mmol/l	
Urate — males	0.12–0.42 mmol/l	
— females	0.12–0.36 mmol/l	
Urea	2.5–6.6 mmol/l	

HAEMATOLOGICAL VALUES

Venous blood: adult reference values

Analyte	Reference values
Bleeding time (Ivy)	Up to 11 min
Body fluid (total)	50% (obese) – 70% (lean) of body weight
Intracellular	30–40% of body weight
Extracellular	20–30% of body weight
Blood volume	
Red cell mass — men	30±5 ml/kg
— women	25±5 m/kg
Plasma volume (both sexes)	45±5 m/kg
Erthrocyte sedimentation rate (Westergren)	0–6 mm in 1 h normal 7–20mm in 1 h doubtful >20mm in 1 h abnormal
Fibrinogen	1.5–4.0 g/l
Folate — serum	2–20 μg/l
— red cell	>100 μg/l
Haemoglobin — men	13–18 g/dl
— women	11.5–16.5 g/dl
Haptoglobin	0.3–2.0 g/l
Leucocytes — adults	4.0–11.0 × 10^9/l
Differential white cell count	
Neutrophil granulocytes	2.5–7.5 × 10^9/l
Lymphocytes	1.0–3.5 × 10^9/l
Monocytes	0.2–0.8 × 10^9/l
Eosinophil granulocytes	0.04–0.4 × 10^9/l
Basophil granulocytes	0.01–0.1 × 10^9/l
Mean corpuscular haemoglobin (MCH)	27–32 pg
Mean corpuscular haemoglobin concentration (MCHC)	30–35 g/dl
Mean corpuscular volume (MCV)	78–98 fl
Packed cell volume (PCV) or haematocrit — men	0.40–0.54
— women	0.35–0.47
Platelets	150–400 × 10^9/l
Prothrombin time	11–15s
Red cell count — men	4.5–6.5 × 10^{12}/l
— women	3.8–5.8 × 10^{12}/l
Red cell life span (mean)	120 days
Red cell life span T (^{51}CR)	25–35 days
Reticulocytes (adults)	10–100 × 10^9/l
Vitamin B_{12} (in serum as cyanocobalamin)	160–925 ng/l

SECTION 1

Your job and its organization

THE HOUSE PHYSICIAN'S DUTIES

The work of the house physician will, naturally, vary from firm to firm and from hospital to hospital, but the following ground rules will usually apply.

Knowing your patients

You should have a good working knowledge of all of your patients: you should know who they are, where in the hospital they are lodged and what the principal diagnoses are in each case. Wherever possible you should see all of your patients each day.

Clerking the patients

You should clerk in as many of your own admissions as possible. Where you take a patient over from another house officer, review the history and examination carefully, re-examining any important items. It is not necessary to re-clerk the patient fully — apart from being a waste of your time, it is irksome for the patient.

Some house officers like to keep a record of every patient under their care in a notebook or a set of file cards. Whichever method you use, a set of brief written notes is essential — do not rely solely on your memory.

Ordering tests and treatment

You will be responsible for ordering blood tests, X-rays, electrocardiograms (ECGs), physiotherapy treatment, etc. on your patients; in many hospitals you will also be expected to take the blood samples. Try to keep a record (preferably in the patient's notes) of which tests you have ordered. When filling out the pathology and X-ray request forms you will find that life is a lot more pleasant if you take the trouble to write legibly and to give a few words of relevant clinical information: a request for a barium enema, for example, is likely to go through without question if you write: 'anaemia, weight loss and lower abdo. pain' in the box marked 'clinical details' but may well be refused if you leave the box blank or write 'hypertension'.

You should make sure that you see and sign all pathology and X-ray reports before they are filed in the notes.

Ward rounds

Before a major ward round, try to ensure that all of the X-ray films and test results are on the ward: cultivate the ward clerk so that he/she will get them for you. During the round you may be expected to write in the notes; make sure that you also make a note in your own notebook of any changes in treatment or tests to be ordered. It is not a good idea to try and fill in request forms during a ward round — this slows the round down, distracts you from whatever else is happening and usually means that the forms are not completed correctly.

Record keeping

Whenever you see a patient, either on your own initiative or because you are called by a nurse, you *must* write something in the notes and the entry must be signed and dated; otherwise others do not know what you have said or done and if your actions are questioned at a later date you will not have a leg to stand on.

Communication

Many complaints made against doctors arise because of poor communications. Do not be afraid of discussing patients' illnesses with them or their relatives in as much detail as is appropriate. (Remember, however, that your ethical duty is to the patient and not to the relatives: it is usually unethical to disclose sensitive information, such as a diagnosis of cancer, to the relatives without telling the patient.)

When you go off duty in the evening or at a week-end you must tell the on-call house physician about any problem patients under your care and any tests needing to be done. If you cannot speak to him/her directly, leave a note pinned to the ward notice board.

Coping with uncertainty

Do not be afraid to ask for advice from your senior house officer (SHO) or registrar or from the nurses — it is far better to ask too often than to struggle on not knowing if you are doing the right thing and feeling more and more inadequate. If you are not getting adequate support from your SHO/registrar, your consultant needs to be told.

THE HOUSE OFFICER'S DAY

Your day is likely to begin somewhere between 8 and 9 a.m. There is much to be said for an early start, especially if you have to do your own blood sampling.

When taking blood samples, lay up a trolley with a tray on top containing needles, syringes, specimen bottles, cotton wool and a tourniquet. Put a 'sharps' bin on the bottom of the trolley. Sort the request forms into sets for each patient. After taking blood from a patient you should *immediately* detach the needle from the syringe and dispose of it in the 'sharps' bin. Label the specimen bottles immediately and put them in the bags or racks with the request forms. At the end of your 'blood round' put the specimens in the appropriate place for collection and dispose of used equipment safely.

Other things which are best done early in the morning include:

- preparing for the ward round, including retrieving X-rays and results and telephoning the laboratory for any 'last minute' results
- getting yourself up to date with any seriously or critically ill patients
- writing discharge prescriptions and discharge letters for any patients who are due to go home that day.

After this you may have to attend a consultant or registrar ward round; if not, you should do a ward round of your own. If any decisions are made about discharge it is as well to write out the discharge prescriptions and discharge letters as early as possible. After the round you may also need to organize special investigations such as computerized tomography (CT) scans (which may require a visit to the X-ray department or a telephone call).

The rest of your day is likely to be taken up with clerking patients, attending clinical meetings, dealing with emergencies or general ward administration. Do not skip clinical or X-ray meetings — remember that the pre-registration year is intended to have an important educational function. Make sure that you get your lunch whenever possible!

At the end of the afternoon the day's crop of pathology and X-ray reports should come back to the ward. Check through them carefully and sign them ready for filing. You may need to make changes to a patient's management on the basis of these results. Write out your request cards for the following morning.

Finally, before you go off duty make sure that your colleague who is on call knows about your problem patients and knows what tests they need to do and what the plans are for treatment.

CONTRACTS AND ENTITLEMENTS

When you start your job you should be offered a formal contract of employment. This not only tells you something about what is required of you; it also formalizes your employment as regards terms and conditions of service, i.e. it protects your rights as an employee. The first rule, therefore, is *read your contract carefully* (however boring it seems) and do not sign it if there are things you are unhappy about or do not understand: discuss them with the personnel officer, a more senior colleague, the mess president, or your local British Medical Association (BMA) representative. The contract should include a specific statement about:

- Your salary.
  The number of Additional Duty Hours (ADHs) for which you will receive payment: these are any hours regularly worked over 40 and relate, therefore, to your on-call hours plus any extras, e.g. being required to come in early or stay late, when you are not on call, for some fixed commitment such as an endoscopy list.
- Leave entitlement.

There should also be a clause stating that the employer cannot make deductions from your salary without your express permission.

Duties

Most contracts are pretty vague in relation to the duties that you will be expected to perform: often they will be said to be 'as set out in the job description'. The job description therefore makes up an important part of the contract, so read that carefully too. As a general rule you cannot be contractually required:

- to work or be on call for more than a total of 83 hours per week (72 hours from April 1994)
- to undertake prospective cover (that is, cover for col leagues who are on holiday or study leave) if to do so would take your average working hours (averaged over the 6 months) to more than 83 hours/72 hours
- to be responsible for private patients (though this may change if you are working for a Trust)
- to work or be on call for a continuous period of more than 56 hours (i.e. a weekend plus the following Monday)
- to be on call without another resident doctor (SHO or registrar) to advise you.

Many contracts or job descriptions also contain a catch-all statement to the effect that 'the practitioner accepts that, in exceptional circumstances, he/she may be required to undertake additional periods of duty to cover for sickness of absent colleagues, etc.' This sounds harsh but is, in fact, just an acknowledgement of reality: if one of your colleagues breaks a leg on the way to work he/she cannot be expected to be on call and, if a locum cannot be found at short notice (see below) you may be asked to do an extra night on call so as to keep the service going.

Entitlements

You are entitled to:

- 13 working days' holiday in 6 months.
- A day off in lieu if you work on a bank holiday. This applies not only to someone who is on duty on the bank holiday itself; it also means that if you are on call on the Sunday before a bank holiday Monday, the hours that you work between midnight and 9 a.m. will entitle you to a day off in lieu.
- A decent, well-furnished room to live in and access to a kitchen and a bathroom — this accommodation is provided free of charge. House officers living in married accommodation are entitled to a rent rebate of up to 25% (50% if both are house officers). The room should contain a cupboard, bedside lamp, easy chair, writing table and telephone (you should not have to leave your room in order to answer your bleep in the middle of the night!).
- There should be regular room cleaning and linen services.

It is very important to book your holiday as far in advance as possible: you cannot be paid for leave not taken and you will not be able to carry more than four days' leave over from one job to the other even if you are working for the same employer.

Locums. Most hospitals nowadays will not employ locums for annual leave but will expect prospective cover to be worked. They should employ locums for sick or other unscheduled leave (e.g. if a member of your family is ill or you are stranded on a Scottish island because of blizzards and cannot get back after your holiday). Even where the hospital employs locums they may not be able to find suitable staff at certain times of year, particularly Christmas, in July or when the Membership of the Royal College of Physicians (MRCP) is being held. Try to give the personnel officer as much notice as possible if a locum is likely to be needed and keep on nagging them if they seem reluctant. Some hospitals say that they will not employ agency locums because of cost: this policy has no basis in NHS guidelines and is almost certainly illegal — if you come across it, consult your mess president or the BMA.

If you work in a teaching hospital a final year student may be appointed as a 'student assistant' to fill in for you when you are away. Such students cannot, however, undertake any on-call duties and are restricted in a number of other ways as regards what they can legally do, so they must not be regarded as being locums in the true sense.

If you find yourself in dispute with the hospital over your contract or about working conditions contact your mess president. If the issue cannot be resolved internally contact your local BMA representative or POWAR (Place Of Work Accredited Representative).

Defence society membership

If legal action is taken against you for negligence or malpractice the hospital will be required to pay for the costs of your defence. You should, however, seriously consider joining the Medical Defence Union (MDU) or the Medical Protection Society (MPS) because:

- The MDU and MPS have vast experience in medical litigation and can give you invaluable advice about how to prepare your statements, how to deal with the solicitor acting for the hospital and a host of other queries. The stress of being involved in litigation is enormous and it is a great relief to be able to rely on sympathetic advice from an expert body.
- The indemnity provided by the hospital does not cover such things as good Samaritan acts or private practice (including cremation forms).

Addresses:

- Medical Defence Union, 3 Devonshire Place, London, W1 2EA. Tel: 071-486-6181
- Medical Protection Society, 50 Hallam Street, London W1N 6DE. Tel: 071-637-0541
- Medical & Dental Defence Union of Scotland, 105 St. Vincent Street, Glasgow G2 5EQ Tel: 041-332-6646.

Tax

Your monthly pay slip will include such things as your tax code and the actual amount of tax deducted at source from your pay. You can reduce your tax liability, quite legally, by claiming for certain expenses incurred in the course of your work: these include the cost of membership of professional bodies such as the BMA or MDU, replacement of medical instruments or damaged clothing. If you wish to claim for these items, ask your local tax office (the personnel department will give you their address) to send you the appropriate forms.

You will also, like all employed persons, be entitled to a single or married person's allowance, i.e. a sum of money on which you do not pay tax. These allowances will be added together and used to create your tax code: thus, if your total of personal allowances is £3500, your tax code will be 350 (i.e. the sum of money minus the last digit). Remember, the higher the tax code, the less tax you pay.

> **When you change jobs be sure to obtain form P45 from your employer, *preferably before you leave the job*. This should be given to your new employer as proof of your tax status; if you do not do this you may end up paying a lot more tax than you should.**

On the other side of the coin, you must declare all earnings from medicine for tax purposes, including things like cremation fees and private earnings.

Other deductions which will be made from your pay include national insurance (simply another form of tax) and superannuation. This is paid into the fund which provides your pension. The superannuation payment should be 6% of your basic salary (not including ADHs).

CONFIDENTIALITY

Hospital medical records are confidential and are the property of the Secretary of State for Health (England and Wales) or a similarly ranking minister in other areas of the UK. Right of access to the notes is usually granted automatically to members of the medical and nursing staff, allied professions (dietitian, physiotherapist, social worker) and to students in those professions. Patients do not have a right of immediate access but, as from 1 November 1991, they can apply to the hospital to see the case notes and such access can only be refused if the consultant in charge of the case considers that disclosure would harm patient's health. If patients ask to see their notes, the most appropriate response is to ask: 'What is it that you want to know?' You can then answer the questions as fully and frankly as you think fit — often a patient just wants to see an X-ray or pathology report. If the patient insists, it is best to hedge (politely) and to refer the question to your consultant.

Certain simple rules will help you to avoid any embarrassing breaches of confidentiality.

- Do not leave notes lying around in public areas of the hospital (e.g. the canteen).
- Do not discuss patients by name in lifts, corridors or stairways where the next-door-neighbour might happen to pass by.
- Do not give information over the telephone to someone claiming to be a relative or close friend unless you have telephoned them to establish identity: confine your remarks to generalities — 'he's a bit better today'.
- When interviewing relatives, be wary of giving sensitive information (e.g. a diagnosis of cancer, poor prognosis, sexually transmitted disease) unless you are sure that the patient is agreeable to your disclosure or that the patient is mentally or physically too enfeebled to give or withhold consent. Remember that your ethical responsibility is to the patient in the first instance, not to the relatives. If the relatives say: 'If it's cancer, I don't want mother to know', you should, politely but firmly, point out that you tell the patients whatever they wish to know and, in particular, that you do not propose to tell the patient a direct lie such as answering the question: 'Is it cancer?' in the negative if the diagnosis is cancer.

CONSENT TO TREATMENT AND CONSENT FORMS

The purpose of asking a patient to sign a consent form is not simply to cover the legal niceties of medical treatment; rather it is to ensure that you explain to the patient in clear and simple language what is to happen to him/her and that you satisfy yourself that the patient understands and feels comfortable with what is to be done.

When is written consent required?

Technically, anything done to a patient (including tapping with a reflex hammer or taking blood) is an assault if performed without the patient's consent. However, implicit consent is assumed for most of these day-to-day, minor interventions. Written consent is required:

- for any operation, even a minor one
- for any investigation which carries a risk of complications (e.g., endoscopy, liver biopsy, arteriography)
- for any form of research.

Table 1.1
The consent form — summary of information required

- Patient's name and address
- A statement that the patient (or the parent or guardian) agrees that the patient will undergo the procedure or operation
- The exact name of the procedure (with side, if appropriate)
- A statement by the patient confirming that the effects of the procedure have been explained to him/her and the name of the doctor who explained them
- A statement by the patient (if he or she so wishes) that certain measures are not consented to (e.g. blood transfusion)
- The patient's signature and the date of signing
- A statement by the doctor confirming that he/she has explained the procedure to the patient
- The doctor's signature and the date of signing

When you go to explain the procedure to the patient and to obtain his/her signature on the consent form, try to pick a time when you will not have to rush. A summary of what the consent form contains is shown in Table 1.1. You should be prepared to mention complications of the procedure (such as haematoma after arterial puncture for angiography) but how fully you explore the subject of complications will obviously vary from patient to patient. If the patient appears at all unhappy about the prospect of complications or the procedure is moderate to high risk (e.g. cerebral angiography) it is wise to:

- ask a more senior person to speak to the patient
- write a full description in the notes of what you have said to the patient.

You cannot obtain valid consent from a patient who:

- has been given a sedative or other drug which interferes with higher mental function
- is under 16 years of age
- is demented.

Note also that the law provides ways in which treatment for psychiatric disease can be given to a mentally incompetent patient without his/her consent; *it does not do the same in respect of treatment for physical disease.* You cannot, therefore, simply ask a relative to sign the consent form. In practice, emergency treatment (such as direct current (DC) cardioversion or laparotomy for appendicitis) is unlikely to result in a prosecution for assault, but in the case of non-emergency procedures you should consult a more senior colleague.

The patient who refuses treatment

Patients have a full legal right to refuse consent to treatment and to take their own discharge from hospital, unless they are deemed to be of such unsound mind that they cannot be allowed to do so (→ below: 'Sectioning'). If patients wish to discharge themselves you should:

- try to persuade the patient to stay and explain to him/her why the investigation or treatment is necessary
- tell the patient that leaving is against medical advice
- ask the patient to sign a self-discharge form (discharge against medical advice form).

Legally, patients are not obliged to sign a self-discharge form and a few refuse to do so. In any case of self discharge, and especially if the patient refuses to sign the form, you must write a full account of events in the notes. You should also, wherever possible, ask a registered nurse to sign the notes as a witness to the truth of your account.

'Sectioning'. Occasional patients become so mentally disturbed that they behave in bizarre and dangerous ways and/or try to discharge themselves when clearly of unsound mind. The Mental Health Act of 1983 provides powers, under Section 5(2), to detain a patient in hospital if he/she is a danger to himself/herself or others and if the condition is urgent. The application must be made on the correct form and requires the signature of a doctor who has seen the patient in the preceding 24 hours *and* of the nearest relative or a social worker.

Normally the medical signature is that of a member of the medical team looking after the patient; the first time you find yourself in this situation, however, you should ask for help from a more senior colleague.

Once you have decided to 'section' a patient, consult the duty psychiatrist for advice about further treatment.

Refusal of specific treatments

Jehovah's Witnesses, Christian Scientists and members of other minority sects may refuse specific treatments such as blood transfusion. You should explain the nature of the treatment to such patients but if it is refused the patients should sign a declaration to that effect. The patients' wishes must then dictate what treatment they receive.

THE NIGHT-ROUND CHECK LIST

To avoid being woken unnecessarily at night, try, some time between 10 p.m. and midnight, to go round the wards for which you are responsible, checking the following:

- Intravenous cannulae (Venflons, etc.): are they working satisfactorily or are they likely to pack up before morning? If in doubt, put in a new one.
- Intravenous infusions: are the i.v. prescriptions written up, with sufficient fluid to last through to the following morning? In the case of small-volume infusions given via syringe drivers (e.g. insulin, heparin), make sure that syringes are loaded, correctly labelled with the patient's name, name of the drug and date and stored in the ward refrigerator.

> It is not reasonable for you to be expected to get up at 3 a.m. to make up drug infusions simply because the nurses on the ward are 'not allowed' or 'not certified' to do it or are not permitted to connect up a solution which you have already made up. If this problem affects you, contact your mess president or BMA representative.

- Night sedation and analgesia: are all those patients who might need these drugs written up for them?
- Beds: does the receiving ward have enough empty beds for emergency admissions? If not, contact your SHO or registrar to arrange transfers of convalescent patients to other wards.
- Sick patients: make sure you have visited all of the very ill patients under your care and done whatever is necessary in the way of either tests or treatment.

DISCHARGING A PATIENT

Ideally, a plan for discharge should be sketched out as soon as a patient is admitted to hospital, so you and the nursing staff should try to assess the likely length of stay and make some provisional plans for discharge. When discharge is imminent, follow the check list below.

- Write your standard letter to the general practitioner: make sure that it includes the name of the consultant, *all* important diagnoses (including chronic conditions like hypertension or diabetes), date of discharge, special home arrangements (e.g. district nurse, home help) and whether the patient will be seen in the out-patient clinic. In special cases, it should also indicate what the patient and/or relatives have been told.
- Where the patient needs a visit from the general practitioner (GP) shortly after discharge or if there have been any special problems it is wise to telephone the GP before discharge.
- Write the prescription for drugs to be taken home, commonly known as TTOs (To Take Out) or TTAs (To Take Away). Whenever possible, try to do this at least 24 hours before discharge. Ensure that the supply is sufficient, particularly if the patient brought in a supply of tablets on admission. Make sure that a copy of this TTO prescription goes to the GP, either on its own or as part of the standard letter.
- Check that the patient knows when and how to take tablets and how to use other devices such as inhalers. (Usually the nursing staff will do this, but you may need to check yourself, especially where inhalers are concerned.)
- Check that any support services have been arranged (district nurse, meals-on-wheels, home help, domiciliary oxygen).
- Check that an out-patient clinic appointment is being arranged.
- Write out request forms for any tests to be done after discharge (e.g. a barium meal or an ultrasound scan).

CERTIFYING DEATH

CONFIRMING DEATH

Check that the patient has no palpable pulse and no audible heart sounds or breath sounds. With patients who have suffered from neurological disease it is wise to check that the pupils are fixed and dilated. Write your observations in the notes and add your signature, the time and the date.

> ⚠ **Do not get involved in confirming brainstem death in a comatose patient. This is a very delicate matter medico-legally and must be done by a senior doctor.**

INFORMING THE RELATIVES

There is no easy way to do this. Try and take a nurse in with you when you meet the relatives, particularly if the patient was relatively young or death was sudden. Try to mention the peaceful nature of the demise or the release from suffering. It is best not to ask for permission for an autopsy immediately after death. If the relatives are not present when death occurs they will usually be telephoned by a senior nurse.

DEATH CERTIFICATE

The death certificate asks you to give your opinion of the cause of death and of any contributory causes. It also asks whether a post-mortem has been or will be held.

Can you issue a death certificate?

You can do so if:

- you have seen the patient alive within 14 days of death *and*
- you are satisfied that death was due to natural causes *and*
- you are reasonably sure of the cause of death.

If you are not sure about the death being a natural one or if you cannot make a reasonable, educated guess at the cause of death, ask a more senior colleague for advice.

If you can issue a death certificate, fill in the appropriate sections, sign and date it; do not forget to fill in the counterfoil in the book.

A few points to remember about filling in death certificates

- 'Cause of death' means the disease or pathological disorder leading to death: it does not mean the mode of dying. Thus coma, cardiac arrest, uraemia, etc. are not causes of death, whereas cerebral haemorrhage, myocardial infarction and hypertensive nephrosclerosis are.
- You do not have to be 100% cast-iron certain of the diagnosis in order to enter it as the cause of death on a death certificate. Thus if you are reasonably confident that a patient died of left ventricular failure due to ischaemic heart disease (IHD) and there is no question of any unnatural cause contributing to death, you can put this down as the cause.

If you cannot issue a certificate

If you did not see the patient before death, another member of the hospital staff may be able to do so. If no-one in the hospital can, the general practitioner may be able to issue a certificate. If you cannot issue a certificate because there is doubt about the nature or cause of death you should discuss the case with the coroner's officer (a police officer). Often, after discussion, the coroner will advise you to go ahead and issue a death certificate; if this is not possible a post-mortem examination or an inquest may be ordered by the coroner. There is space on the back of the death certificate to notify the registrar that you have discussed the case with the coroner but in practice you will hardly ever have to fill this in. In particular, it is *not* wise to do so if you have discussed the case with the coroner and have been advised to issue a certificate, as filling in the box will delay the funeral arrangements.

CONSENT FOR A HOSPITAL POST-MORTEM

Doctors often wish to have a hospital autopsy for their own education and interest; this is quite separate from autopsies ordered by the coroner. You may ask permission of the relatives for a hospital post-mortem only if you have already decided to issue a death certificate: what you cannot legally do is to ask the relatives' permission and then, if they refuse, refer the case to the coroner. Try to obtain consent on the morning after the patient's death, not immediately they have died, and emphasize the educational value to yourself and colleagues. Stress that the body will be treated respectfully and that the relatives can, if they wish, state that they do not wish for a particular part (usually the head and neck) to be examined. If you are filling in the death certificate before you have spoken to the relatives and you intend to ask for permission for a post-mortem, you should indicate this on the certificate. If permission is subsequently refused, the registrar will get to know about it eventually, so no harm is done.

WHOM TO INFORM ABOUT A DEATH

Poor communications in this area can lead to long-lasting bitterness and resentment, so make sure that the following are informed as soon as possible:

- the relatives
- the GP (it is quite in order for the ward clerk or a nurse to do this, so long as it is done)
- the team looking after the patient (if not your own team)
- your consultant (if it is one of your own team's patients).

MEDICO-LEGAL PROBLEMS

It is as well to be aware right at the outset that medical practice has become increasingly hedged in with legal problems and dangers. You must understand that *no-one is immune* — however good a doctor you are and no matter how much your actions may have been in good faith, you may still find yourself hauled before a court if you are unlucky or make a simple (though understandable) mistake. The commonest legal pitfalls can be considered under several headings (→ also other chapters on confidentiality (→ p 9) and on prescribing controlled drugs (→ p172)).

Note-keeping

Medical defence societies will tell you that they are often unable to defend an action against a doctor, not because he/she has done wrong but because they cannot establish from the notes that the right things were done at the right time. You must, therefore:

- write legible, complete notes, preferably using an ink that will not fade and which will photocopy well
- sign and date your entries in the notes and make sure that your signature is legible or is accompanied by a printed rendering of your name
- avoid slang and any abusive or sarcastic remarks, either relating to the patient or to any other doctors involved in the case.

It is also advisable to state in the notes what the plan of management is so that it is clear that you have thought about the problems and are trying to do the best for the patient.

Disclosure of information to third parties

You must not discuss details of a patient's illness or treatment with anyone without his/her permission. If a close relative asks about the patient there is usually no problem over providing simple information, especially face to face (→ below). However, if the information is in any way sensitive you may need to withold it, at least until you are sure that the patient is willing for it to be disclosed: remember that, ethically, your 'contract' is with the patient, not the relatives.

Telephone enquiries. If you receive a telephone call from someone who is apparently the relative of a patient, do not say anything specific but confine your remarks to generalities such as 'He's had a better day today' or 'She's quite comfortable at the moment'. If the caller is very anxious to know more (e.g. if he/she is a long way away and wants to know if an urgent trip to the hospital is necessary) offer to ring the caller back and, in the meantime, ask the patient's permission to discuss details of his/her condition with the caller. In general, full discussions about a person's illness are much better conducted by asking the relative to come into the ward at a mutually convenient time.

Press and media enquiries. It is extremely easy to say the wrong thing under questioning from an experienced journalist. In almost all cases it is best to say nothing to the media but to refer all enquiries to your boss or to an official hospital spokesperson.

Police enquiries. The police may ask you to give them information about a patient in connection with the investigation of a crime or a potential prosecution. You should tactfully point out that you cannot release privileged information to them except with the patient's permission: ethically it is much better to say nothing, even if that means that the patient escapes prosecution for a minor offence. Where the offence in question is a serious one, however, (such as murder, rape, arson or terrorism) you may feel that your duty as a citizen overrides your duty as a doctor; certainly, in such a case a court is unlikely to rule against you if you find yourself being sued for breach of confidence.

Communication

Failure on the part of doctors to keep each other informed is a major cause of ill-feeling between colleagues and also of medico-legal hazards. When you go off duty, make sure that you have told your colleague who is on call about any seriously ill patients under your care; similarly, when you have been on call you must tell other firms about any of their patients who have been admitted during the night or to whom you have been called.

Communication with nursing staff is also important; your life can be made a misery if you ignore this principle. Do not go off for your half day without telling the nurses and do not turn your bleep off when on call. Make sure that any instructions you write for them (such as i.v. fluid prescriptions) are clear, sensible and will last through the night. Finally, remember communication with the GP: tell him/her immediately if a patient dies (→ p 17) and make sure that the note you write for the GP when a patient is discharged is legible and clear, especially in relation to take-home drugs.

Prescribing

The prescribing of controlled drugs is dealt with on page 172. Many of the cases which occupy the energies of the medical defence societies are, however, related to the prescribing of ordinary, everyday drugs. Be especially careful with:

- drugs which commonly cause allergy (e.g. penicillin)
- drug interactions, especially with chemically promiscuous substances such as warfarin

- dilutions, e.g. of cardiovascular drugs like dopamine/dobutamine; check your arithmetic carefully, especially in the middle of the night.

Fitness to drive

People with certain medical conditions may be partially or completely unfit to drive: such restrictions can apply to people with epilepsy, diabetes, angina, strokes, syncopal attacks, etc. The regulations are especially severe for holders of vocational licences (Large Goods Vehicles and Passenger Carrying Vehicles). Full details of these regulations can be found in the 'red book', *Medical Aspects of Fitness to Drive*, which should be available in your hospital library. A brief summary of the most important regulations is given in Table 1.2.

Table 1.2
Regulations for fitness to drive

Condition	Regulation
Epilepsy	Cannot drive unless he/she has been free of fits for 2 years or has had fits only during sleep for 3 years. Note that a fit which occurs *for any reason* (including missed medication) will result in a driving ban. Vocational driving is forbidden if someone has had a fit after the age of 5 years
Myocardial infarction (MI)	May not drive for 2 months after the event
Angina	Should not drive if angina is easily provoked by driving. *Note:* people with ischaemic heart disease of any kind are almost always banned from holding a vocational licence
Complete heart block	Driving is forbidden until 1 month after the fitting of a pacemaker. Vocational licences may not be held, even when a pacemaker has been fitted
Syncopal attacks	May not drive until the cause has been established and treated effectively
Diabetes	No restriction if treated by diet alone and has normal vision. Treatment with tablets or insulin usually restricts licence to a 3-year term. Vocational licences cannot be held if patient treated with insulin
Stroke	Should not drive for at least a month, longer in more severe cases (e.g. those with a hemianopia). Rules for vocational driving will depend on individual case

Note that the responsibility for informing the Driving and Vehicle Licensing Centre (DVLC) about a medical condition which may affect driving rests with the patient, not the doctor. Patients should be warned, however, that they risk prosecution if they knowingly withhold information about a serious medical disorder.

HUMAN IMMUNODEFICIENCY VIRUS (HIV) TESTING

People at risk of HIV infection

The HIV virus is of relatively low infectivity and is, therefore, transmitted by intimate contact or by blood-borne transmission; it cannot be passed on by casual non-intimate contact such as shaking hands, sharing towels, crockery, etc., social kissing or being in a confined space with an infected person. There is a risk of infection from:

- penetrative sexual intercourse (vaginal, anal or oral if the recipient partner has an open lesion in the mouth or on the lips)
- sharing needles or syringes to inject drugs
- receiving contaminated blood products via a transfusion (now a very rare cause of infection in the UK but may be a risk for those travelling abroad, e.g. to East Africa)
- vertical transmission from mother to baby.

Testing patients

If a patient asks for an HIV test you should try to establish:

1. Why a test has been asked for. Has there been true at-risk behaviour or does the patient have a misconception about how HIV is transmitted?
2. When did the at-risk behaviour take place? Remember that it can take up to 3 months for the HIV antibody to become detectable after infection has occurred, so a negative test within that time does not rule out infection.
3. What does the patient hope to learn from the test. The test does not detect acquired immunodeficiency syndrome (AIDS) nor does it predict, for those who are positive, who will develop AIDS or how long it will be before they do so.
4. What will the patient do if the result is positive? Try to ask a specific question such as: 'What support will you have' or 'What will be your greatest concern' rather than a very general one such as: 'How will you feel?'.

If you are unhappy with the responses to any of these questions ask someone more senior to see the patient. You should also explain that, if the test is positive, there are organizations who will provide counselling and support, often on an urgent basis. On the negative side, having an HIV test can have certain disadvantages; for example, most life assurance companies ask if a proposer has been HIV tested or has sought counselling in relation to HIV. If the answer to the question is yes, insurance (and, therefore, such things as mortgages) may be refused, or granted only at increased premium, even if the result of the HIV test itself was negative.

Surgical or other invasive treatment

There are very few circumstances in which it is necessary to obtain the result of an HIV test as an emergency. If the at-risk patient needs elective surgery the question of HIV status should have been sorted out well in advance. If, on the other hand, emergency surgery is needed then it should be assumed that the patient is HIV positive and management should be on that basis. If one of your seniors objects, try pointing out that a negative test would not in any way be reassuring: if the person has been indulging in high-risk behaviour within the last 3 months, he/she might be infected and yet test negative. The only safe thing to do is to assume that people with a history of high-risk behaviour are HIV positive.

Transplant donors

An ethical difficulty arises in relation to persons who are brain-dead and are suitable to be organ donors for transplantation: most transplant centres require that donors be tested for various infections, including HIV. You should, ideally, explain this to the relatives when permission is being sought for the use of the brain-dead person's organs. It is worth spending a moment thinking about what will be said if the HIV test proves to be positive: if there are no implications for the health of others (for example if the donor is unmarried or has not had a sexual partner for many years) then the relatives may not wish to know the result of the test and you should not force it upon them. If, however, there are potential health hazards involving other people then someone needs to discuss this with the family once the result is known. This job is best delegated to your SHO, registrar or consultant.

Positive test results

Patients who have a positive test, need to be interviewed (not necessarily by you) so that the significance of the result can be explained. Point out again that the test is not a test for AIDS and that it cannot predict when (if ever) the person will develop AIDS, though the great majority of HIV-positive individuals do eventually develop the disease. Try to put patients in touch with a counsellor, either locally via an AIDS helpline or via one of the national charities such as the Terence Higgins Trust.

Negative test results

You should again emphasize that the result does not definitely exclude infection and that it certainly does not sanction unsafe behaviour such as unprotected sex or sharing needles. If the patient is in doubt, most hospitals now have a counselling service which can provide leaflets to educate patients about safe behaviour.

Nursing HIV-positive patients

HIV is of low infectivity and there is no need for these patients to be isolated unless they have some other indication such as diarrhoea. Staff with cuts or open wounds on the hands should not handle vomitus, urine, faeces, etc. from HIV-infected patients — indeed, anyone handling such material should wear gloves. You should also wear gloves when taking blood from an HIV-positive patient and take extreme care over sharps disposal.

> **If you prick yourself with a needle after taking blood from an HIV-positive person, contact the microbiology department (or the Consultant in Communicable Disease Control) immediately.**

POTENTIAL ORGAN DONORS

Many patients in the UK die or suffer prolonged dependency because of a lack of organs for transplantation. Therefore, all doctors should consider organ donation in any young or middle-aged patient with a fatal condition whose kidneys, liver, heart or corneas are healthy.

Suitable organ donors

- Victims of severe head injury
- Severe sub-arachnoid or intra-cerebral haemorrhage
- In the case of corneal donation, any young patient with healthy eyes and a rapidly fatal illness.

Unsuitable organ donors

- Where brain death is uncertain (→ below)
- Those over 60
- Where there has been significant hypotension or hypoxia during the final illness
- Where there is a history of previous disease affecting the potential donor organ (e.g. hypertension or diabetes in the case of kidneys or hepatitis B or alcohol abuse in the case of the liver)
- Where the patient has received drug or other treatment which might have affected the organs to be transplanted
- In the case of kidneys, where there is persistent oliguria.

Diagnosis of brain death

This is a complex area and you should not attempt to make this diagnosis yourself: it requires the involvement of a senior doctor. However, there is no point in even considering brain death if the following apply:

- the patient is able to breathe spontaneously
- the coma might be due to drugs, poisoning or a metabolic disorder such as uraemia
- the patient has easily-elicitable brain stem reflexes such as pupil reactions, gag reflex.

Potential organ donors

- Talk to the relatives (UK law does not allow the removal of organs without the consent of the next of kin, even if the patient was carrying a donor card). It is best to interview the relatives in the company of a senior nurse and, preferably, not in the middle of the night. Try to put across the point that a tragedy has already occurred and that one way for some good to come out of it is for the organs to be used for transplantation.

Many families are helped by being told that they can receive information later about the person who has received their loved ones' organs, a practice which many transplant surgeons will undertake.

- You will need to explain to the family that, as a matter of routine, all potential organ donors are tested for the presence of infections, including HIV. Ask the family whether they wish to be told the results of the HIV test and *write their reply in the notes*.
- Talk to a senior member of your firm; raise the question of establishing the diagnosis of brainstem death.
- Discuss with your senior colleagues the question of contacting your local transplant co-ordinator or the nearest transplant centre.
- While waiting for a decision about organ donation or for the organs to be removed, make sure that the potential donor is kept supplied with adequate fluid and that blood pressure is maintained.
- The transplant centre will ask you to carry out tests on the potential donor such as hepatitis B and HIV testing and HLA determination. As regards HIV tests, you should ask the family if they wish to be told the result (→ above). If a potential donor is found to be HIV positive, this will have implications for spouse, children and sexual partners, so tell your consultant and leave it to him/her to take the matter further.

SECTION 2

Clinical problem solving

WEIGHT LOSS

Causes (→ Table 2.1)

Table 2.1
Causes of weight loss

Common	Diabetes mellitus Malignancy Thyrotoxicosis Depression Anorexia nervosa AIDS Malabsorption: Coeliac disease Pancreatic insufficiency Blind loop syndrome Chronic ill health leading to depression of appetite, e.g. uraemia
Uncommon	Tuberculosis Adrenal insufficiency Oesophageal stricture

The commoner causes of weight loss will be somewhat different in the older as compared to the younger subject: thus, in an older patient malignancy would be more prominent as a cause of weight loss but AIDS less so; social and geographical factors are also important. Assessing patients' weight in relation to their height is often useful: this can be calculated as the body mass index (BMI):

$$\text{BMI} = \frac{\text{Weight (kilos)}}{(\text{Height [meters]})^2}$$

The normal range for BMI is 20–25 for a male, 19–24 for a female.

History

Ask about:

- thirst and polyuria
- mood (the patient with anorexia nervosa typically says that everything is fine and, in particular, does not complain of weight loss)
- heat or cold intolerance
- symptoms of organ-specific disease, e.g. cough, sputum, breathlessness, pain
- dysphagia, vomiting, diarrhoea and steatorrhoea.

Examination

General systemic abnormalities should be carefully sought, e.g:

- anaemia
- clubbing
- lymphadenopathy
- skin rashes.

Other points to note in the examination are:

- to check for signs of thyrotoxicosis
- to check for an abdominal mass, especially the liver or spleen
- to remember to look for signs of endocarditis in any susceptible patient
- to look out for signs of i.v. drug abuse.

It is important to do a dipstick urine test for glucose.

Investigations

Apart from those indicated by the history and examination, the following should be considered:

- full blood count (FBC) and film
- biochemical profile, including liver function tests (LFTs)
- blood glucose
- thyroid function tests
- chest X-ray (CXR)
- blood cultures in patients with a pyrexia.

Patients who might have AIDS must be nursed as if HIV positive until the results of serology are known (→ also p 25).

FEVER

Fever is commonly (but not invariably) caused by infection and infection, if present, may be bacterial, viral, protozoal, fungal, etc. Therefore the golden rules for dealing with a febrile patient are:

- **Do** attempt to find out the cause of the fever by means of a proper history and examination.
- **Do** take proper samples for culture and for serology and make sure they are properly stored.
- **Do not** give a febrile patient antibiotics without a diagnosis unless he/she is seriously ill.
- **Do not**, in adults, give an antipyretic unless the patient is extremely uncomfortable because of the fever. You will simply confuse the issue.

Remember that a low-grade pyrexia (less than 38°C) is often normal in patients who are receiving a blood transfusion or in the first 24 hours after an operation; there is no need to do anything in such cases unless the patient is unwell.

DIAGNOSIS OF THE CAUSE OF FEVER

History

It is obviously wise to ask initially about symptoms related to the common fevers, i.e. sore throat, cough, sputum, dysuria, pain in any site, diarrhoea, purulent discharge. If the patient is febrile on admission you should also ask about weight loss, night sweats (a feature of lymphomas and tuberculosis), foreign travel, contact with infectious disease or animals, recent medication, appearance of a rash.

Examination

First assess how ill the patient looks, to check for the presence of a rash and to note other general pointers such as lymphadenopathy, clubbing, splinter haemorrhages. Remember to check any i.v. infusion sites to make sure that the patient does not have phlebitis or cellulitis. It is also important to:

- examine the mouth and throat
- examine the heart (checking especially for signs of heart failure and for new murmurs)
- examine the lungs
- check any sites of pain
- check for signs of deep vein thrombosis (DVT) if the patient has been bed-bound.

Investigation

In any patient with a significant fever (sustained temperature above 38°C) you should:

- perform a full blood count
- take blood for blood cultures
- do a dipstick test on the urine to check for protein and blood
- depending on the history and examination, send off samples of urine, sputum, stool, throat swab, etc. for culture
- arrange a CXR
- if myocardial infarction (MI) or pulmonary embolism (PE) is suspected, do an ECG
- take blood for viral serology
- if there is a history of foreign travel, take blood for thick and thin film examination for malaria.

Immunocompromised patients. In patients who are known to be neutropaenic (white cell count less than $2 \times 10^9/l$) or to have AIDS, infections can progress rapidly and be extremely serious or even fatal; the same is true in patients with advanced chronic renal failure or (to a lesser extent) diabetes. Therefore, episodes of fever in such patients should be assessed as a matter or urgency and treated aggressively. If an immunocompromised patient becomes febrile, you should go through the routine described above but, in addition, take blood for culture from any central venous lines or Hickman lines. Make sure you inform a more senior member of your team if an immunocompromised patient becomes febrile.

MANAGEMENT

If the patient is well and the fever is only mild (less than 38°C) it is wise not to treat until a firm diagnosis has been made. If the patient is poorly or the temperature is higher than 38°C, treatment should be based on the most likely clinical diagnosis. The British National Formulary (BNF) gives guidance on the use of antibiotics in specific circumstances; a summary of the recommendations is given below (p 230). You should also check with your local hospital formulary which might make slightly different recommendations from those in the BNF.

LYMPH NODE ENLARGEMENT

Minor lymph node enlargement is common in certain circumstances, for example in children with upper respiratory infections and in the inguinal nodes of many adults.

CHECKING FOR LYMPHADENOPATHY

You should check specifically for lymph node enlargement in the following circumstances:

- unexplained fever or weight loss
- persistent cough or shortness of breath
- unexplained anaemia or bruising
- patients who are jaundiced
- patients with finger clubbing
- suspected breast cancer
- increased risk of TB, e.g. immigrants, socially deprived, homeless, alcoholics, those who are HIV positive.

UNEXPECTED LYMPHADENOPATHY

History

Review the history, asking specifically about:

- weight loss
- respiratory symptoms
- abnormal bleeding and bruising
- infections in the relevant area
- contact with unusual infections, e.g. farm animals (brucellosis), domestic animals (toxoplasmosis)
- risk factors for HIV infection.

Examination

- If the enlarged nodes are in the neck, check the head and neck carefully, including the mouth and throat.
- Check for finger clubbing.
- In women, be sure to check for breast lumps.
- Examine the chest for signs of reduced movement, consolidation, pleural effusions or a fixed rhonchus (a sign of bronchial obstruction).
- Examine for abdominal masses, especially the liver and spleen.

Investigations

- Virtually every patient with lymphadenopathy should have a blood count and erythrocyte sedimentation rate (ESR), LFTs and a CXR.
- If an infectious cause is suspected, ask for a glandular fever screening test and appropriate serology, e.g. brucella, toxoplasma.

- If tuberculosis (TB) is suspected, obtain sputum for smear and culture and early morning urines (the *whole* of the specimen passed first thing in the morning) for culture. A tuberculin test (Mantoux or Heaf test) may be useful, especially by excluding TB if the test is negative.
- If there is a pleural effusion a diagnostic aspiration should be performed: withdraw 20 ml of fluid using a standard venepuncture needle and syringe and send the sample to the laboratory for cytology, protein concentration, culture and sensitivity.

> Fluid specimens for cytology must be sent to the laboratory fresh. The cells will be unrecognizable if the sample is stored in the refrigerator overnight.

- A pleural biopsy may be needed. Consult your SHO or registrar.
- Aspiration cytology or biopsy of an enlarged lymph node may be required. Consult your SHO or registrar.

ANAEMIA

Although anaemia has many causes, the most common in the UK in adults are:

- iron deficiency due to menstrual losses with inadequate replacement
- iron deficiency due to a colonic carcinoma
- anaemia of chronic disease (e.g. rheumatoid arthritis, cancer, chronic inflammation)
- oesophagitis secondary to a hiatus hernia.

> Peptic ulcer is an uncommon cause of anaemia as such, though it is of course a common cause of haematemesis.

Other important but less common causes of anaemia include gastric carcinoma, pernicious anaemia, bone marrow dyscrasias (aplastic anaemia, leukaemia, etc.), blood loss due to inflammatory bowel disease, malabsorption (especially coeliac disease), chronic renal failure. Dietary deficiency is a rare cause of anaemia in Britain (though common elsewhere), as are haemolytic diseases and haemoglobinopathies.

History

- Take a detailed menstrual history in any woman of reproductive years or who is within 2 years of the menopause.
- Ask about abdominal pain.
- Ask about bowel habit and changes in habit, also about the character of the stool.
- Ask about appetite, nausea and vomiting.

Examination

Look especially for evidence of weight loss or abnormal bruising. Check for lymphadenopathy. In the abdomen, check for enlargement of liver or spleen and for any masses. Make sure to perform a rectal examination. It is *negligent* to fail to do this.

Investigations

Full blood count and ESR. A low mean corpuscular volume (MCV) usually indicates iron deficiency, a high MCV may suggest B_{12} or folate deficiency but can also occur with liver disease, alcohol abuse, hypothyroidism and occasionally in other circumstances such as haemolytic states. The blood count and film may give a clue to other diagnoses such as haemolysis or leukaemia. The ESR will show a progressive rise with greater degrees of anaemia but very high values (over 100) suggest a collagen-vascular disease (think of temporal arteritis/ polymyalgia rheumatica in older patients) or malignancy.

Haematinics. Send samples for:

- serum iron and total iron-binding capacity (TIBC) or (preferably) ferritin
- serum B_{12} and folate
- red cell folate.

If haemolysis is suspected, send blood for LFTs, reticulocyte count, haptoglobins and Coombs' test. If a haemoglobinopathy is suspected, ask for HbA_2 and F, sickle test and Hb electrophoresis. It is also wise to discuss the case with your local haematologist.

Radiology. A barium enema is essential in any patient who might have a colonic carcinoma; prior to the X-ray a sigmoidoscopy should be performed to check the lowest 10 cm of the rectum to ensure that there is not a stenosing lesion which would render a barium enema dangerous. If available, colonoscopy is a suitable alternative to sigmoidoscopy and barium enema. If malabsorption or Crohn's disease is suspected, a small bowel meal or small bowel enema might be appropriate. Discuss the exact requirement with the X-ray department or a more senior colleague.

> ⚠ **All men over 50 and all post-menopausal women, if presenting with unexplained anaemia, have a carcinoma of the colon until proved otherwise.**

Endoscopy. This is the preferred method for investigating the upper gastrointestinal (GI) tract. It is at least as accurate as radiology and allows lesions to be biopsied. In older patients, beware of attributing the anaemia to peptic ulceration or oesophagitis. These may well co-exist with a more sinister lesion in the colon.

Biopsy. Request an endoscopic small bowel (usually duodenal) biopsy if coeliac disease is suspected. Aspiration and/or biopsy of bone marrow is indicated in suspected pernicious anaemia or bone marrow dyscrasias. If you are unsure whether there is an indication for bone marrow examination in a particular case, ask your local haematologist.

Other tests. In suspected pernicious anaemia or in a patient with B_{12} deficiency of unknown cause, a test of B_{12} absorption, such as a Schilling test, is required. You should also ask for an auto-antibody screen with particular reference to gastric parietal cells, intrinsic factor and thyroid antigens.

Management

This will depend on the underlying cause: it is rarely possible to justify blood transfusion without a diagnosis of the cause of the anaemia.

Iron. This should almost always be given orally and usually as ferrous sulphate tablets. Side-effects such as abdominal discomfort and constipation are dose-related so that the precise formulation is unimportant; however, a once-daily preparation may be useful in the elderly to aid compliance, while in those who have trouble swallowing tablets, a syrup may be prescribed. Treatment should continue until the haemoglobin level is normal and for about 3 months thereafter to replenish body iron stores. Where a patient is severely intolerant of oral iron or compliance is a major problem, a total-dose intravenous infusion may be given. This must be undertaken with care, beginning with a test dose, and under medical supervision with facilities to hand to treat anaphylaxis (see BNF).

The Hb does not rise any more quickly after intravenous iron than with oral iron therapy.

Vitamin B_{12}. This is given intramuscularly in a dose of 1 mg of hydroxocobalamin every 2 to 3 days to a total of 5 mg, followed by 1 mg every 3 months.

In a patient with severe B_{12}-deficiency anaemia the myocardium is abnormal due to a sort of 'B_{12}-deficient cardiomyopathy'; when treatment with B_{12} is started the serum potassium will fall rapidly, so regular measurements of serum potassium, and supplements of potassium, are essential.

Folic acid. This is given orally, usually in a dose of 5 mg t.d.s. If a patient has, or might have, B_{12} deficiency as well as folate deficiency, he/she *must* be given a dose of vitamin B_{12} before starting folic acid, to avoid possible neurological complications of B_{12} deficiency.

Blood transfusion. (→ also p 163) In the treatment of anaemia, as distinct from acute blood loss, transfusion is indicated if the patient has symptoms from his/her anaemia or the Hb is less than 8 g/dl. You should take all necessary blood samples for investigations before transfusing the patient. Replacement of blood should normally be with packed red cells, aiming to bring the Hb level up to around 10 g/dl. Each unit of blood will raise the Hb level by about 1 g/dl. In the elderly or in someone with heart failure, give 20 mg of frusemide with each unit of packed cells in order to avoid fluid overload. Patients with pernicious anaemia should not be transfused as they are very sensitive to fluid overloading and because transfusion may cause the bone marrow to 'shut down'. In chronic renal failure, transfusion is not usually necessary unless the Hb is less than 7 g/dl and also carries a high risk of fluid overload. Consult a more senior colleague.

CHEST PAINS

Chest pain is a common symptom, the cause of which may be serious. The most important features of the pain, so far as making a diagnosis is concerned, are:

- What type of pain is it? Patients are not always good at describing pain so it is worth offering the patient a list of choices, e.g. burning, stabbing, crushing, pulling.

> Beware of the patient who says he/she has a 'sharp-pain'. Patients often describe a pain as 'sharp' when they mean that it is severe.

- Where is the pain and is it localized or more diffuse?
- Does the pain radiate to a distant site?
- Is the pain affected by breathing or movement?
- Are there any associated symptoms such as shortness of breath, nausea or faintness?

SERIOUS CAUSES

The commonest serious causes of chest pain are: angina, MI, PE, pericarditis, pleurisy, pneumothorax, aortic dissection and malignant infiltration.

Angina

Clinical features. This is usually a heavy or crushing pain in the centre of the chest radiating to one or both arms (especially the left), the neck or the jaw. It is sometimes described as sharp and is usually brought on by exertion or emotion. Left-sided pain alone, especially if localized to a small area under the left breast (without radiation), is usually not angina. Relief by glyceryl trinitrate (GTN) supports a diagnosis of angina but may also occur if the pain is due to oesophageal spasm.

Myocardial infarction (MI)

Clinical features. This pain is like that of angina but is said to be more severe and is often accompanied by sweating, faintness, shortness of breath or nausea; occasionally patients feel that death is imminent. Cardiac pain lasting for more than 20–30 min is likely to be due to infarction rather than angina; in practice, however, the distinction is often impossible.

Examination. This may be normal but look especially for:
- pallor, sweating, degree of distress
- tachycardia
- hypotension
- chest wall tenderness (usually mild if it is cardiac pain)
- gallop rhythm

- signs of pulmonary oedema
- pericardial friction rub (occasionally).

Investigation. The most important investigation in suspected angina/MI is an ECG; indeed, you must request an ECG in anyone who might have ischaemic cardiac pain even if you think other diagnoses are more likely. An ECG done during pain is particularly helpful. Examples of ECGs showing the changes of MI/acute ischaemia are given in Figures 5.1–5.4, (→ p 219).

Remember in the early stages of an MI the ECG may be normal.

Management. If you think that an MI is very probable or strongly possible, you should arrange urgent transfer to a coronary care unit (CCU). Give analgesia (usually diamorphine, 5 mg i.v. with prochlorperazine 12.5 mg), oxygen and (if breathless) intravenous frusemide (40 mg) before transfer and make sure that an intravenous cannula is in place before leaving the general ward or accident and emergency (A&E) department. If no bed is available on the CCU, arrange a bedside cardiac monitor and ask the nursing staff to check pulse and blood pressure (BP) every half hour. Treatment with a thrombolytic agent or with inotropic drugs (dobutamine, milrinone, enoximone) may need to be considered: for this and other reasons you should inform the duty medical registrar (→ p 219).

If a patient complains of angina-type pain which has been coming on more frequently, lasting longer and provoked by lesser degrees of exertion but the initial ECG is normal, the diagnosis may be crescendo angina (unstable angina); this can be diagnosed more confidently in someone with a long history of stable angina (months or years).

The treatment for unstable angina consists of:

- bed rest with cardiac monitoring
- beta-blockade (unless contraindicated)
- aspirin (unless contraindicated)
- nitrates (oral or intravenous)
- calcium antagonists
- intravenous heparin in severe cases.

Serial ECG and cardiac enzymes tests should be requested to exclude an MI.

Unstable angina carries a high risk of progression to MI. If the pain cannot easily be controlled with simple treatment, consider i.v. nitrates by infusion and i.v. heparin. In a patient who fails to settle quickly on such treatment and who might in general terms be a candidate for coronary artery surgery or angioplasty, you should discuss the management with a cardiologist.

Pulmonary embolism (PE)

Clinical features. In the case of a small or medium-sized embolism the pain is well localized, often severe and knife-like and accompanied by shortness of breath and considerable distress. There may be haemoptysis. When the embolism is large the pain is often central and accompanied by faintness, collapse and hypotension.

Examination. This may be normal but you should look especially for:

- pallor or cyanosis
- a raised jugular venous pressure (JVP) without peripheral oedema
- tachycardia
- hypotension
- an area of dullness in the chest with crackles, bronchial breathing or a pleural friction rub
- a gallop rhythm.

Investigation. *Do not forget to check the legs for evidence of a DVT.* If you suspect a PE you should ask for a CXR and ECG (but remember that a normal CXR and ECG do not exclude the diagnosis). It is also worth checking the arterial blood gases (ABGs). Typically someone with a significant PE will have a reduced PaO_2 and $PaCO_2$.

Management. Treatment of PE consists of anticoagulation, pain relief and oxygen. Anticoagulation is usually started with heparin, 5000 U as an i.v. bolus followed by an infusion of about 1000 U per hour, the dose being adjusted so as to keep the partial thromboplastin time (activated partial thromboplastin time: APTT; kaolin cephalin clotting time: KCCT) two to three times the control. Subcutaneous heparin (standard or low molecular weight forms) might be used in some units. Warfarin is introduced within the first few days (regimes vary). Oxygen should be given, provided there is no contraindication, at whatever concentration is needed to maintain a PaO_2 above 8.0 kPa and preferably above 10 kPa. Analgesia can be given by mouth or, if the pain is more severe, by intramuscular or intravenous injection; opiates are often necessary.

> **If a patient with a suspected PE is hypotensive or shocked, you are faced with a grave emergency → p 53 and contact your SHO or registrar immediately.**

Pericarditis

Clinical features. The pain resembles angina but is more definitely made worse by breathing. There is often a tachycardia and there may also be a pericardial friction rub.

Examination. The ECG may show sinus tachycardia and widespread ST segment elevation.

Management. Treatment is with analgesics; non-steroidal anti-inflammatory drugs (NSAIDs) such as naproxen or indomethacin are often effective. Ask the nursing staff to carry out regular observations of pulse and BP – some patients with pericarditis will develop a pericardial effusion or tamponade.

Pleurisy

Clinical features. This is rare nowadays as an isolated phenomenon but often accompanies lobar pneumonia. There is usually a history of several hours to several days of malaise, cough, fever, shortness of breath and pleuritic-type chest pain (i.e. localized and markedly exacerbated by deep breathing or coughing). The onset may be surprisingly sudden (mimicking a PE). Ask about recent foreign travel. Legionnaire's disease is common in some favourite holiday spots and can cause lobar pneumonia.

Examination. Physical examination may reveal fever, reduced chest movement on the affected side, tachycardia and an area of dullness with crackles or a pleural friction rub. The CXR typically shows an area of dense, uniform opacification corresponding to one or more lobes.

Management. Treatment consists of antibiotics, analgesia, rehydration and oxygen and physiotherapy as required.

Pneumothorax

Clinical features. This occurs in two major groups of patients: firstly the young, fit, asthenic person and secondly the middle-aged or elderly person with chronic obstructive lung disease, chiefly emphysema. Pneumothorax may also complicate acute asthma. The pain usually begins very abruptly and may be felt over an area of the chest wall or over the shoulder. The patient may say that 'something seemed to snap and then the pain and shortness of breath suddenly began'. The pain is usually pleuritic. Dyspnoea can vary from mild to very severe depending on the size of the pneumothorax and whether there is tension within it or not. Physical signs are often absent but if the pneumothorax is large there may be hyperresonance on the affected side together with reduced breath sounds. In the case of a tension pneumothorax the patient is often very breathless, pale and cyanosed and the trachea may be displaced to the opposite side. In such a case more senior help should be sought urgently.

Investigation. This consists of CXRs taken in inspiration (the standard view) and expiration (to show evidence of a small pneumothorax); blood gas analysis is helpful if the patient is very symptomatic.

Management. Treatment of small pneumothoraces consists of analgesia and rest with a repeat CXR the next day. If the pneumothorax is larger (more than 33% of the area of the hemithorax) treatment should be by aspiration or tube drainage (→ p 130). If there is tension the pneumothorax must be aspirated as an emergency.

Aortic dissection

This condition is uncommon but, when it occurs, has a high mortality. The pain may mimic that of MI or it may begin in, or radiate to, the interscapular area. Patients often describe the pain as tearing or pulling in nature and say that it gets relentlessly worse over an hour or two after its onset. Physical signs are often absent but you should look for inequality of brachial and radial pulses between the two sides, inequality of blood pressure readings between the two arms and evidence of an aortic diastolic murmur.

Investigation. The ECG may be normal or may show changes suggesting acute MI. The most helpful routine investigation is the CXR which typically shows widening of the mediastinal shadow.

Management. This should begin with a 'phone call to your SHO or registrar. The patient should be given adequate analgesia (usually diamorphine) and oxygen. The BP must be lowered to minimize the risk of extension of the dissection and agitated patients should be given sedation.

> **The BP should be lowered to a level below 120 mmHg systolic, using intravenous labetalol, hydrallazine or nitroprusside if necessary.**
>
> - **Urgent investigation to confirm the diagnosis and to assess the extent of the dissection is desirable: echocardiography and CT scanning of the chest are the investigations of choice.**
> - **If a dissection is suspected, your SHO or registrar should ring the on-call team at the nearest cardiac surgical unit.**
> - **Anticoagulants and thrombolytic agents are absolutely contraindicated.**

Maligant infiltration of the chest wall and ribs

Clinical features. Pain from this cause is usually of longer duration. It often has a boring or deep aching quality, keeps the patient awake at night and is affected to a varying degree by respiration. The most likely malignancies to produce this disorder are carcinomas of the bronchus or breast, myeloma and mesothelioma.

Examination. This may reveal local chest wall tenderness or signs of a pleural effusion. There may also be evidence of disease elsewhere such as clubbing, lymphadenopathy or an enlarged liver. *Remember to examine the breasts in women.*

Investigation. This will vary according to the probable underlying cause but is likely to include blood count, ESR, LFTs, rib X-rays, bone scan and aspiration of any associated pleural effusion.

LESS SERIOUS CAUSES

Less serious causes of chest pain include: reflux oesophagitis or gastritis, oesophageal spasm, benign chest wall pain and herpes zoster.

Reflux oesophagitis or gastritis

Clinical features. The pain does not usually radiate to the arms (though it may to the back). It bears no relation to exercise and typically has a burning or squeezing quality. There may be a history of previous indigestion. The pain may, in the past, have been brought on by bending, stooping or lying flat. It is relieved by antacids.

Examination. This is usually negative though there may be some tenderness in the epigastrium.

Management. Treatment is with antacids and reassurance.

Oesophageal spasm

Clinical features. This can sound very like angina but does not radiate to the arms and is not exercise-related. It may be relieved by nitrates or calcium antagonists. Differentiation from cardiac pain can sometimes be made by considering other risk factors (age, family history, smoking history, gender); in some cases it requires an exercise test or other cardiac investigations.

Management. Treatment is by reassurance and the use of nitrates, calcium antagonists, H_2-receptor antagonists or motility agents such as metoclopramide.

Benign chest wall pain

Clinical features. This may result from musculoskeletal strain and typically gives rise to pain following exertion which is localized to a small area of the chest and is accompanied by chest wall tenderness. Tietze's syndrome is a particular form of chest wall pain in which the patient feels sudden, intense pain in a very small area of the chest wall which remits after 2-3 seconds. The cause is unknown.

Herpes zoster

Clinical features. Pain in the distribution of one or two intercostal nerves may appear before the rash. Typically the pain is unpleasant, hot and burning or pricking in nature and affected only slightly if at all by respiration. It is usually followed within 1–3 days by the characteristic erythematous, vesicular rash.

Management. Treatment with oral acyclovir, if given very early (within 24 hours of the appearance of the rash) may abort an attack.

HYPERTENSION

Hypertension may be defined as a blood pressure consistently above 140/95. It may present a problem to the house physician in one of three ways:

- a patient is admitted electively for investigation and treatment of known hypertension
- a patient is admitted as an emergency for treatment of severe hypertension or its complications (left ventricular failure, visual disturbance, renal failure, hypertensive encephalopathy, aortic dissection)
- discovered in the course of managing a patient with a related condition (stroke, MI) or an unrelated one.

GENUINE HYPERTENSION

If hypertension has not been diagnosed before, it is important to measure the BP yourself and to see several readings over 2 or 3 days before coming to a decision. The only exception to this is if the BP is very high (over 200 systolic or 120 diastolic) *and* is definitely causing acute complications such as papilloedema, fits, left ventricular failure (LVF), renal failure or aortic dissection.

UNDERLYING CAUSES

Usually there are none, but it is obviously worth looking for one.

History

Ask about:

- personal or family history of renal disease
- previous history of hypertension, e.g. during pregnancy
- symptoms which might suggest a phaeochromocytoma, e.g. palpitations, headache, attacks of pallor.

Examination

- In patients under 40, check the femoral pulses for radio-femoral delay.
- Examine the heart for cardiomegaly and for 3rd or 4th heart sounds.
- Examine the chest for evidence of left ventricular failure.
- Examine the abdomen for renal masses and bruits.
- Examine the optic fundi for arteriovenous nipping (significant only in patients under 65), exudates, haemorrhages and papilloedema. If you find retinopathy this indicates that the hypertension has been present for months or years rather than coming on acutely.
- Finally, be on the lookout for signs of Cushing's syn-

drome, e.g. central obesity, livid striae in the skin, thinning of skin over the hands, moon face, proximal myopathy.

Investigations

- Every patient with hypertension should have the urine examined for casts, protein and blood.
- Take blood for urea and electrolytes (U&E); if there is proteinuria or oedema, ask for a serum albumin.

> A low serum potassium in someone who has not been taking diuretics, particularly if accompanied by a raised bicarbonate, should make you think of Conn's syndrome.

- Ask for an ECG and chest X-ray to look for evidence of left ventricular hypertrophy and strain and of left ventricular failure.
- In patients under 50 you should consider the possibility of a phaeochromocytoma, so send off two 24-hour urine samples for vanillylmandelic acid (VMA).

> A high proportion of patients with phaeochromocytoma have sustained hypertension, not intermittent as is often suggested in textbooks.

- In younger patients or where there is a suggestive history, renal function should be investigated by means of an isotope renogram or intravenous urogram (IVU) (renal ultrasound is not sufficient as you need to know about function and not just structure).

MANAGEMENT

Non-urgent treatment

Your chief may have a particular favourite drug or drugs for treating hypertension. If not, consider using the following:

Thiazide diuretics. These are effective both at reducing BP and at lessening the risks of hypertension-associated diseases. They do not reduce BP very much so are suitable only for patients with mild to moderate hypertension (180/110 or less).

Beta-blockers. They reduce BP and are particularly suitable for patients who also have angina; they may be combined with diuretics. They should be used *with great caution, if at all,* in patients with peripheral vascular disease and are contraindicated in patients with a history of airways obstruction or heart block. Beta-blockers must not be used alone in patients suspected of having a phaeochromocytoma, who require combined alpha- and beta-blockade.

Angiotensin converting enzyme (ACE) inhibitors. These have a good side-effect profile and often need to be taken only once daily. They are particularly useful in patients with associated heart failure. ACE inhibitors can cause worsening of renal function in the presence of renal artery stenosis and renal function should be carefully monitored (at least every 48 h) after an ACE inhibitor has been introduced. This is especially true of patients who have widespread atherosclerotic vascular disease, in whom clinically silent renal artery stenosis is common. ACE inhibitors may cause first-dose hypotension, especially in patients who have been taking diuretics so the first dose should be given with the patient lying in bed and BP should be measured every 10 to 15 min for the first 2 hours.

Calcium antagonists. These also have a good side-effect profile and are useful in people with angina. Verapamil should not be used in people who have, or who are at risk of, heart failure and should only be combined with a beta-blocker *with great caution.*

Non-drug methods of controlling BP. These should not be forgotten, especially weight reduction and reducing alcohol consumption.

Urgent treatment

> ⚠ **It is nearly always more dangerous to reduce BP rapidly than to leave it untreated or to reduce it slowly.**

The best treatment for a hypertensive emergency can be selected from Table 2.2.

Table 2.2
Treatment for hypertensive emergency

Type of emergency	Drug of choice	Drug to avoid
Encephalopathy	Sodium nitroprusside, labetalol, diazoxide	Beta-blockers, clonidine, methyldopa
Cerebral haemorrhage or infarction	Sodium nitroprusside, labetalol	Beta-blockers, clonidine, methyldopa
Myocardial ischaemia or infarction	Nitrates, labetalol, calcium antagonist sodium nitroprusside	Hydralazine, diazoxide, minoxidil
Acute pulmonary oedema	Sodium nitroprusside, plus loop diuretics, nitrate plus loop diuretic	Hydralazine, diazoxide, beta-blockers, labetalol
Aortic dissection	Sodium nitroprusside, plus beta-blocker, labetalol	Hydralazine, diazoxide, minoxidil
Acute renal failure	Sodium nitroprusside, labetalol, calcium antagonist	Beta-blockers
Grade III or IV retinopathy	Sodium nitroprusside, labetalol, calcium antagonists	Beta-blockers, methyldopa, clonidine
Microangiopathic haemolytic anaemia	Sodium nitroprusside, labetalol, calcium antagonists	Beta-blockers

LOW BLOOD PRESSURE

As with most measurements in medicine, it is the change in blood pressure which is more significant than the absolute value: an elderly man whose BP is usually 170/100 but who suddenly drops down to 110/70 is likely to need further investigation. Remember also that, at least in advanced societies, average BP rises progressively with age, so a reading of 95/50 might be quite normal in a 17-year-old girl but would not be at all normal in a middle-aged subject.

Hypotension impairs vital organ function by:

- reducing coronary perfusion
- reducing renal blood flow and therefore urine output
- reducing cerebral perfusion and thereby impairing consciousness.

Causes

The three principal causes of hypotension are summarized in Table 2.3.

Table 2.3
Causes of hypotension

Diagnosis	Cause
Volume depletion:	
Blood loss	(gastrointestinal, trauma, into a fracture, leaking aortic aneurysm)
Loss of crystalloid or colloid	e.g. from diarrhoea, vomiting, loss from drains, diabetic ketoacidosis, burns, polyuric renal failure, over-vigorous use of diuretics
Pump failure:	
MI	
Major arrhythmias	fast atrial fibrillation (AF), supra ventricular tachycardia (SVT), ventricular tachycardia, complete heart block
Pulmonary embolism (large)	
Myocardial depression due to septicaemia or acidosis	
Myocardial depressant drugs	e.g. beta-blockers, anti-arrhythmics
Over-vigorous treatment of hypertension	
Excessive fall in peripheral vascular resistance	
Septicaemia	
Peritonitis	
Pancreatitis	

> **Uncommon but important causes include adrenal insufficiency, self-poisoning with drugs, e.g. phenothiazines or antidepressants, tension pneumothorax, aortic dissection, pericardial effusion (tamponade), anaphylaxis.**

Gynaecological causes such as rupture of an ectopic pregnancy should be considered in appropriate patients.

DIAGNOSIS

History

1. Ask about:

- pain (chest, abdominal or back)
- breathlessness
- any indications of blood loss, especially melaena. In young women, ask about the date of the last period.

2. Review the drug history. Could there be a pharmacological cause?

Examination

1. Remember to check the following:

- Does the patient look dehydrated?
- Is the patient cold, clammy and peripherally shut down?
- Does the patient look as though he is suffering?
- Is the patient fully conscious?
- Is the patient pyrexial?
- Is the JVP visibly distended or collapsed?
- Is the patient sweating?

2. Check the patient's pulse and BP yourself. Measure the BP with the patient supine and also sitting upright: a fall in systolic pressure of 30 mmHg or more (or a fall to less than 90 mm) makes it likely that the patient is volume depleted.

3. Examine the heart, looking for a gallop rhythm, pericardial friction rub, new murmurs. If the patient has interscapular pain (which is suggestive of an aortic dissection) check both carotid and both brachial pulses to look for inequality of pulse volume.

4. Examine the respiratory system, looking for reduced chest movement on one side, tracheal deviation (both of these would occur with a tension pneumothorax), markedly reduced breath sounds, a pleural rub (which would suggest pulmonary embolism).

5. Examine the abdomen, looking for evidence of peritonitis or ileus and for an aortic aneurysm; if you suspect leakage from an aneurysm make sure you check the femoral pulses.

6. Check any drains for evidence of bleeding and be sure to perform a rectal examination if gastrointestinal bleeding is suspected.

INVESTIGATIONS AND MANAGEMENT

Volume depletion

Suspected bleeding. Take blood for full blood count, U & E and blood grouping. Losses should be replaced as whole blood; concentrated red cells should only be used in frail or elderly patients where there is a major risk of overload from over-transfusion. Insert a urinary catheter to monitor urine output.

Other causes of fluid loss. Take blood for FBC and U & E, then give intravenous fluids such as plasma expanders (Gelofusin, Haemaccel, etc.) or saline. If the loss seems to be of water more than solutes, i.e. if the patient is dry as the result of poor drinking or perspiration, the i.v. fluid of choice is 5% glucose. Remember, however, that water depletion rarely results in hypotension of more than mild degree. (For a fuller discussion of intravenous fluid therapy, → p 153). Insert a urinary catheter to monitor urine output.

> ➘ When treating hypovolaemia remember the possible risk of overloading the patient with fluid; if you are at all concerned about this a central venous line should be put in to monitor central venous pressure (CVP).

Pump failure

Arrange an ECG and look for:

- tachycardia
- rhythm disorder or heart block
- pathological Q waves, ST segment elevation and other evidence of MI
- signs of PE, namely, right axis deviation and deep, slurred S waves in lead I, QRS widening in V1, V2, ST segment depression and T wave inversion in V1 and V2.

If you are not sure how to interpret the ECG ask the duty medical registrar.

Arrange a CXR to look for:

- pneumothorax
- pulmonary oedema
- collapse or consolidation
- widening of the mediastinum (aortic dissection).

Myocardial infarction (MI). Urgent transfer to a CCU is indicated. Give analgesia (usually diamorphine, 5 mg i.v. with prochlorperazine 12.5 mg), oxygen and (if breathless) intravenous frusemide (40 mg) before transfer and make sure that the patient has an intravenous cannula in place before he/she leaves the general ward or A&E department. If no bed is available on the CCU, arrange a bedside cardiac monitor and ask the nursing staff to check pulse and BP every half hour. Treatment with a thrombolytic agent or with inotropic drugs (dobutamine, milrinone, enoximone) may need to be considered: for this and other reasons you should inform the duty medical registrar.

Rapid tachycardia (over 140 per min). This may be a compensatory reaction to the volume depletion but a tachyarrhythmia should also be considered, so look at the ECG and, if in doubt, ask for help with interpretation. If you are *sure* that the rhythm is an SVT, then provided the patient is not in pulmonary oedema and has not recently been given a beta-blocker it would be reasonable to attach the patient to a cardiac monitor and to give verapamil, 5 mg i.v. over 2 minutes, repeated if necessary.

Large pulmonary embolism (PE). Give 60% oxygen (28% in a patient with a previous history of obstructive airways disease) and analgesia where required. Further treatment lies between heparinization, streptokinase and urgent cardiac surgery. Make sure the patient is receiving plenty of i.v. fluid so as to increase right ventricular filling (and hopefully, therefore, right ventricular output) and commence i.v. heparin, 5000 units stat followed by 10 000 units over 8 h via an infusion pump, then ask for help.

Dissection of the thoracic aorta. Give analgesia and, if the patient is distressed, a sedative. Contact your registrar urgently: he or she should speak to the duty surgical registrar at your nearest cardiac surgical centre.

Fall in systemic vascular resistance (SVR)

Fluid replacement. The patient with an abnormally low SVR of whatever cause is, in effect, fluid depleted, so give fluid in the form of colloid solutions, i.e. albumin, Gelofusin, Haemaccel or hetastarch.

Septicaemia. Think about possible infective foci and send off appropriate samples for culture; do blood cultures in any case and send off a coagulation screen (platelet count, prothrombin time, partial thromboplastin time and fibrinogen titre or D-dimer). These will be abnormal if the septicaemia has given rise to disseminated intravascular coagulation (consumption coagulopathy). Check FBC, U & E and ABG.

Pending the results of blood gas estimation, give 60% oxygen (28% if the patient has a history of obstructive airways disease). Septicaemic patients are severely ill, so fluid balance and throughput should be monitored by inserting a central venous pressure line and a urinary catheter.

Once blood and other cultures have been taken the patient should be commenced on intravenous broad-spectrum antibiotics such as a cephalosporin (cefuroxime, cefotaxime, etc.), Augmentin, gentamicin, ciprofloxacin, Primaxin. If you are not sure which to use, ask. In patients with evidence of disseminated intravascular coagulation (DIC) fresh frozen plasma(FFP) maybe needed (to replace clotting factors) or platelets.

Sepsis may result in myocardial depression so if the patient remains hypotensive despite having a normal central venous pressure, consider using an inotropic agent (dobutamine, milrinone, enoximone). If urine output is poor despite a normal CVP, consider low-dose dopamine infusion; this drug *must not* be given into a peripheral vein.

Corticosteroids, often in high doses, have been extensively used in the treatment of septicaemic shock but recent research has shown that they are of no value.

Pancreatitis. Check serum amylase: a level higher than 1000 is diagnostic, while one over 500 is highly suggestive. Take blood for FBC, U & E, glucose and calcium. Management consists of fluid replacement and analgesia; proteinase inhibitors such as aprotinin (Trasylol) are of no value and urgent surgery is rarely necessary.

Perforation of a viscus. Arrange chest and abdominal X-rays. The patient may need urgent surgery or re-operation (if the problem arises postoperatively).

Miscellaneous

Tension pneumothorax. A large-bore needle should be inserted into the second intercostal space in the mid-clavicular line. This often results in a dramatic improvement in the patient's clinical condition. You should then insert a chest drain (→ p 132).

Adrenal insufficiency. If you are really stuck for an explanation for the hypotension, consider this: take a blood sample to be stored for later estimation of serum cortisol and give i.v. hydrocortisone, 100 – 200 mg stat (depending on the size of the patient) then 100 mg every 6 h, together with intravenous 0.9% saline.

HAEMOPTYSIS

Causes (→ Table 2.4)

Table 2.4
Causes of haemoptysis (in order of frequency)

Small haemoptysis	PE Pneumonia Carcinoma of the lung Pulmonary oedema ENT causes (nose or pharynx)
Large haemoptysis	Bronchial carcinoma PE Bronchiectasis TB Lung cavity (e.g. mycetoma)

History

First make sure that the patient is actually describing haemoptysis and not haematemesis: try to see a specimen of sputum if possible. Haemoptysis is usually bright red and may be frothy whereas haematemesis is more likely to be granular and reddish-brown.
Ask about:

- chest pain
- breathlessness
- purulent sputum
- weight loss
- past history of chest disease and heart disease.

Examination

- Look at the patient generally for evidence of anaemia, finger clubbing, lymphadenopathy and cachexia.
- Examine the heart and chest fully, looking for asymmetry of chest movement, deviation of the trachea, cardiac murmurs, signs of pulmonary oedema and signs of lobar consolidation. Listen for a pleural friction rub.
- Examine the abdomen for hepatomegaly (carcinoma or TB).
- Examine the legs for signs of a DVT.

Investigations

The key investigation is a CXR (postero-anterior, PA, and lateral). You should also ask for sputum to be sent for culture (1 specimen), cytology (3 specimens) and, where appropriate, tubercle bacilli. You should also consider an FBC, LFTs and ECG.

Management

According to the underlying cause.

BREATHLESSNESS

It is useful to subdivide causes of breathlessness into acute (coming on within minutes or hours) and sub-acute or chronic (coming on over days or weeks) (→ Tables 2.5, 2.6).

Table 2.5
Causes of acute dyspnoea (in order of frequency)

Pulmonary oedema
- LVF
- Mitral valve disease

Bronchopneumonia (including exacerbations of chronic bronchitis)
Asthma
PE
Lobar pneumonia (especially pneumococcal)
Pneumothorax
Extrinsic allergic alveolitis
Psychogenic

Table 2.6
Causes of sub-acute dyspnoea (in order of frequency)

Chronic bronchitis
Pulmonary oedema
- Left ventricular failure
- Mitral valve disease

Asthma
Bronchopneumonia
Anaemia
Lobar pneumonia
Pleural effusion
Carcinoma of the lung
Recurrent pulmonary embolism
Pericardial effusion
Fibrosing alveolitis

FIRST STEPS

If you are telephoned by a ward to tell you that a patient is breathless, try to find out:

- over what length of time the dyspnoea has come on
- how ill the patient is (e.g. is there any clouding of consciousness?)
- the bedside observations, i.e. pulse, BP, temperature and respiratory rate
- associated symptoms such as chest pain, cough, sputum, wheezing, haemoptysis.

HISTORY

Ask about:

- how severe the dyspnoea is, i.e. whether it occurs at rest as well as on exertion
- the time scale
- associated symptoms as above
- any previous history of chest disease.

An audible wheeze. Ask about a past history of asthma, whether there are pets at home, any history of occupational exposure to allergens. Review the drug history with particular reference to beta-blockers and NSAIDs.

Lobar pneumonia. If the patient has a fever and localized, pleuritic chest pain, ask about foreign travel and contact with infectious disease.

EXAMINATION

You should perform a full cardiovascular and respiratory examination, including pulse rate, respiratory rate and BP. A few important points to remember:

- A person can be hypoxic without being cyanosed.
- Tachypnoea is an important physical sign, especially in the elderly, where it may be the first sign of bronchopneumonia (before there is any fever).

> **In a patient with asthma: pallor, exhaustion, tachycardia, inability to speak more than one or two words, quiet breath sounds are all signs of *severe asthma* (→ p 224).**

- In cases of PE, a pleural rub is the exception rather than the rule; it is more useful to check for a raised JVP and a gallop rhythm. Many cases of PE have no physical signs.

INVESTIGATIONS

Acute dyspnoea

- Hb and white cell count
- CXR (if you suspect a pneumothorax, ask for both an inspiratory and an expiratory film)
- ECG (for suspected MI, PE or heart failure).

More than mild dyspnoea. Check ABG. An arterial PO_2 of less than 8 kPa (60 mmHg) indicates severe hypoxaemia. Consult your SHO or registrar.

Febrile patients. Blood and sputum cultures should be performed.

Suspected PE. Check the KCCT (APTT). Arrange a ventilation/perfusion lung scan as soon as possible.

Sub-acute dyspnoea

- Hb and white cell count
- CXR
- ECG
- sputum culture
- sputum for cytology (if a carcinoma is suspected)
- ABG at rest and after exercise.

Asthma. Consider an eosinophil count, IgE and radio allergosorbent test (RAST) to look for specific allergens.

Suspected extrinsic allergic alveolitis. Send blood for avian precipitins and precipitins against aspergillus and other fungi.

Consider requesting spirometry or fuller lung function tests, with transfer factor.

MANAGEMENT – ACUTE DYSPNOEA

Pulmonary oedema

1. Establish an i.v. line and give frusemide, 50 mg as a bolus. Consider giving regular i.v. diuretics.
2. Give oxygen by face mask. If a venturi-type mask is to be used, give 10 l per min. If there is a previous history of chest disease, give 4 l per min.
3. Give diamorphine, 5 mg i.v.
4. If the condition is severe, give isosorbide dinitrate by intravenous infusion, 5 mg per hour (increased to 10 mg per hour if needed).
5. If the patient is in fast atrial fibrillation, check serum potassium; once you know that the serum potassium is above 4.0 mmol/l, give digoxin, 0.5–0.75 mg by i.v. infusion in 100 ml of 5% glucose (*not* saline) over 20 min. If the patient has some other form of tachyarrhythmia this may need urgent treatment: consult your SHO or registrar.
6. If the patient is hypotensive (systolic BP less than 100 mmHg), consider i.v. dobutamine infusion.
7. Consider (CVP) monitoring and urinary catheterization.

Bronchopneumonia (e.g. exacerbation of chronic bronchitis)

1. Give nebulized salbutamol, 2.5 – 5 mg every 4 to 6 h, depending on the severity of the condition.

2. Give oxygen, 24% (2 l per min) if there is a previous history of chronic obstructive airways disease, otherwise 40% (10 l per min).
3. Having taken blood and sputum cultures, give antibiotic in the form of ampicillin, 500 mg every 6 h or amoxycillin, 500 mg every 8 h. If the patient is allergic to penicillin, give trimethoprim, 200 mg every 12 h or tetracycline (oral dose: 250 mg every 6 h; i.v. dose: 500 mg every 12 h).
4. If the patient has a lot of tenacious sputum, arrange chest physiotherapy.
5. If the patient is very breathless despite nebulized salbutamol, add nebulized ipratropium bromide (Atrovent), 250 – 500 µg four times daily.
6. Consider an oral theophylline or, if the patient is very breathless despite nebulized bronchodilators, aminophylline by i.v. infusion: dilute aminophylline 500 mg in 500 ml of 5% glucose or 0.9% saline. The rate of infusion will depend on whether the patient has been taking an oral theophylline before admission or not, and on his/her size. *If the patient has not been taking an oral theophylline at home,* give i.v. aminophylline as follows:
   Small patient .... 600 – 1000 ml/24 h
   Medium-sized patient .... 900 – 1500 ml/24 h
   Large patient .... 1100 – 2000 ml/24 h

   If the patient has been taking an oral theophylline at home, take blood for measurement of theophylline level, then give i.v. aminophylline at half the above rate.
7. Give hydrocortisone, 100 mg i.v. followed by a second dose 6 h later. If the patient can swallow, start oral prednisolone, 30 – 40 mg once daily in the morning.

Pulmonary embolism (PE)

1. Give oxygen, 24% (2 l per min) if there is a previous history of chronic obstructive airways disease, otherwise 40 – 60% (10 – 12 l per min).
2. Having checked the KCCT (APTT), give a bolus dose of heparin, 5000 u i.v. followed by an infusion at a rate of

17 500 u per 12 h. Re-check KCCT (APTT) after 10 hours' treatment and adjust heparin dose accordingly (→ Table 2.7).

3. Give pain relief as needed. Do not be afraid to give diamorphine if the pain is severe.

Table 2.7
Heparin infusion schedule

Loading dose	5000 iu i.v. over 5 min
Initial infusion rate	25 000 iu heparin made up in saline to 50 ml gives a final concentration of 500 iu/ml, to be started at 2.8 ml/h (1400 iu/h)

Check APTT at 6 h. Adjust according to APTT ratio (APTT: control) as follows:

APTT ratio	*Infusion rate change*
> 7	stop for 30 min to 1 h and reduce by 500 iu/h
5.1–7.0	reduce by 500 iu/h
4.1–5.0	reduce by 300 iu/h
3.1–4.0	reduce by 100 iu/h
2.6–3.0	reduce by 50 iu/h
1.5–2.5	no change
1.2–1.4	increase by 200 iu/h
< 1.2	increase by 400 iu/h

4. If the lung scan confirms the diagnosis, start warfarin: check prothrombin time (PT), then give a dose of 10 mg warfarin and repeat the PT 18 h later. Give subsequent doses of warfarin according to Table 2.8.

Table 2.8
Warfarin schedule*

Day	International normalized ratio (INR) (9–11a.m.)	Warfarin dose (mg) given at 5-7 p.m.
1st	< 1.4	10
2nd	< 1.8	10
	1.8	1
	> 1.8	0.5
3rd	< 2.0	10
	2.0–2.1	5
	2.2–3.2	4.5
	2.4–2.5	4
	2.6–2.7	3.5
	2.8–2.9	3
	3.0–3.1	2.5
	3.2–3.3	2
	3.4	1.5
	3.5	1
	3.6–4.0	0.5
	> 4.0	0
		Predicted maintenance dose
4th	< 1.4	> 8
	1.4	8
	1.5	7.5
	1.6-1.7	7
	1.8	6.5
	1.9	6
	2.0–2.1	5.5
	2.2–2.3	5
	2.4–2.6	4.5
	2.7–3.0	4
	3.1–3.5	3.5
	3.6–4.0	3
	4.1–4.5	Miss out next day's dose, then give 2 mg
	> 4.5	Miss out 2 days' doses, then give 1 mg

* Suggested warfarin schedule based on INR. Modified from Fennerty et al. *British Medical Journal* 1988; 297: 1285–8.

APTT should be within or below therapeutic range (1.5-2.5 times control). If APTT is above this range the heparin effect on INR should be neutralized by adding protamine (0.4 mg/ml plasma) to the sample.

If the lung scan is equivocal but the clinical suspicion of PE is strong, consider bilateral venography.

5. If the patient is shocked, give plasma expander and consider streptokinase. *Ask for help from a more senior person.*
6. Have the patient fitted with anti-embolism stockings.
7. Consider investigating the patient for a thrombotic tendency, especially if the thromboembolism is recurrent or if the pulmonary embolism is large.

Asthma

The management of asthma is discussed more fully on pages 224–227. As a general rule, patients who are ill enough to need admission for their asthma should be treated aggressively with nebulized or i.v. bronchodilators and with steroids.

Lobar pneumonia

1. Give antibiotics in the form of benzylpenicillin 1.2 g 6 hourly i.v. (plus erythromycin 1 g 6 hourly i.v. if the pneumonia is severe). If the patient is penicillin-allergic, give erythromycin as above or cefuroxime, (750 mg i.v. 6 hourly). If an 'atypical' pneumonia (*Mycoplasma* or *Legionella*) is possible, take blood for viral studies (which usually includes these organisms) or for specific *Mycoplasma* and *Legionella* serology, then give erythromycin, 1 g 6 hourly i.v.

In early pneumococcal pneumonia, the most useful investigation for identifying the organism is blood culture.

If the patient is known to have AIDS or if this is a strong possibility, the pneumonia could be due to *Pneumocystis carinii.* This will require treatment with high-dose co-trimoxazole or pentamidine : *consult your SHO or registrar.*

2. Give analgesia as required if there is pleuritic pain. Do not be afraid to use opiates if these appear necessary.
3. If the PaO_2 is less than 10 kPa (75 mmHg) give oxygen, 40% (10 l/min) unless there is a previous history of chronic obstructive airways disease, in which case you should give 24% (2 l/min).

Pneumothorax

If the pneumothorax is small (just a rim of air around the lung) and the patient is not significantly breathless, no treatment is required other than analgesia and observation. If the pneumothorax is larger or the patient is very breathless then aspiration or formal drainage will be needed (→ p 130).

If you think the patient has a *tension pneumothorax* (indicated by severe dyspnoea and an obvious shift of the mediastrium to one side), ask your SHO or registrar for urgent help : a large bore (18-gauge) needle should be inserted into the second intercostal space in the mid-clavicular line. If your SHO/registrar cannot come immediately you should put the needle in yourself. Once the tension has been relieved the patient will need a chest drain.

Psychogenic dyspnoea

Be wary of making this diagnosis unless the patient is known to be hysterical or very neurotic or there is a past history of a similar episode. In severe cases the patient will breathe deeply and rapidly and may complain of peri-oral tingling or paraesthesiae in the hands. As the condition progresses there may be carpopedal spasm or even loss of consciousness. Treatment is by encouraging patients to re-breathe their own expired air using a large paper bag. Once the acute attack is over a psychiatric assessment and/or sedative drugs may be indicated.

MANAGEMENT: SUB-ACUTE OR CHRONIC DYSPNOEA

Chronic bronchitis

In mild cases the patient may require nothing more than a bronchodilator inhaler for intermittent use. Most older people, however, are not very good at using a traditional metered-dose inhaler and do better with a breath-actuated inhaler (Aerolin Auto-haler) or a dry powder inhaler (Ventolin Rotahaler or Bricanyl Turbo-haler). In more severe cases, especially where reversible airways obstruction can be demonstrated on spirometry, the patient may benefit from a steroid inhaler such as Aero-Bec, Becotide Rota-haler, Pulmicort Turbo-haler or (if the patient prefers) Becotide or Becloforte inhaler. An oral theophylline (e.g. Uniphyllin, Phyllocontin Continus, Slo-Phyllin, etc.) is often useful, particularly where nocturnal breathlessness is a problem.

> ↘ Treatment of patients taking oral theophyllines should be monitored by measurements of plasma theophylline concentrations. The level should be maintained between 10 and 20 mg/l (55–110 μmol/l).

Left ventricular failure (LVF)

Once the acute episode is over the patient may be adequately treated with a small dose of diuretic, e.g. frusemide, 40 mg once or twice daily; this is often combined with a potassium-sparing diuretic in a compound tablet such as Frumil, Frusene or Burinex A. If, however, the dose of diuretic required is more than 80 mg of frusemide per day (2 mg bumetanide per day) it is often appropriate to treat the patient with an ACE inhibitor (→ p 178). After starting an ACE inhibitor the patient's U & E should be checked every second or third day. Because ACE inhibitors cause potassium retention there is usually no need to give a potassium-sparing diuretic: frusemide (or bumetanide) alone should be used.

Asthma (→ also p 224)

Once the patient is recovering to a point where he/she is almost ready to come off nebulized bronchodilators (usually the peak flow rate will be above 300 l/min), start inhaled steroids and an inhaled $beta_2$-adrenergic agonist. *Check that the patient is able to use his/her inhalers properly.* Talk to the patient about how to tail off oral steroids and about measuring his/her own peak flow rates at home. Some patients may require inhaled cromoglycate or an oral theophylline.

Pleural effusion

Symptomatic relief can often be achieved by aspirating a pleural effusion. You should observe the procedure on one or two occasions before doing it yourself and should be supervised during your first few attempts (→ p 128).

Pericardial effusion

If moderately large or very large this may require aspiration, which must be done by a senior person, so consult your SHO or registrar.

ABDOMINAL PAIN

Those patients who are admitted as an emergency because of abdominal pain will usually come under the care of a surgical team. However, you should be aware of the problem of abdominal pain in 'medical' patients, either as an accompaniment to the admission diagnosis or occurring during a stay on a medical ward.

Causes (→ Table 2.9 and 2.10)

Table 2.9
Causes of abdominal pain accompanying an acute 'medical' diagnosis

Common	Alcoholic gastritis Gastroenteritis Food poisoning Peptic ulcer Pancreatitis (in a patient admitted with a fever of unknown cause or with jaundice) Inflammatory bowel disease (IBD) (especially Crohn's disease) MI Basal pneumonia (may simulate gallbladder disease) Mesenteric embolism (especially in a patient with AF, a recent MI or severe heart failure)
Rarities	Diabetic ketoacidosis Sickle cell crisis Herpes zoster Henoch-Schönlein purpura Porphyria

A word of caution: a patient with a 'medical' condition and abdominal pain is quite entitled to have more than one diagnosis, so do not be too ready to attribute the pain to the medical disorder.

Table 2.10 **Causes of abdominal pain arising de novo in medical in-patients**	
Non-serious causes	Gastritis Constipation Urinary tract infection (UTI) Irritable bowel syndrome
Serious causes	Any cause of an "acute abdomen", but especially: • Mesenteric embolism (in a patient with AF, a recent MI or severe heart failure) • Leaking aortic aneurysm (in someone with known arterial disease) • Pancreatitis (in a known alcohol abuser or someone with biliary disease)

Clinical assessment

You will obviously need to take a proper history and carry out an appropriate examination. Try to answer the following questions specifically:

- Is the patient shocked?
- Is there any evidence of peritonism?

If you are considering urinary tract infection (UTI), make sure that the urine is dip-stick tested as soon as possible, then send a midstream specimen of urine (MSSU) to the laboratory.

Investigations

If the cause of the pain appears potentially serious, ask for an FBC and U & E. If there is a possibility of pancreatitis, ask for a serum amylase. If the patient has known heart disease *or* the pain might be due to cardiac causes *or* the patient might have to go to theatre *or* the patient is shocked, arrange an urgent ECG. If the patient is shocked or has evidence of peritonism, your SHO or registrar needs to be informed immediately. In such a case, arrange an X-ray, of the chest (erect) and of the abdomen (erect and supine).

Management

This will depend on the cause, but certain general principles apply.

1. Keep the patient nil by mouth.
2. Ask the nurses to perform half-hourly pulse and BP.
3. If the patient is shocked, take blood for a coagulation screen and for 'grouping and save' and resuscitate with intra-

venous fluids (usually a colloid such as Haemaccel or Gelofusin).

4. If the patient is systemically ill, is shocked or has signs of peritonism, involve your SHO or registrar at an early stage. You may also need an urgent surgical opinion.

VOMITING

Causes

There are many possible causes of vomiting, most of which are quite common, so keep an open mind(→ Table 2.11).

Table 2.11
Causes of vomiting

Gastrointestinal	Hiatus hernia, oesophageal stricture, oesophageal carcinoma, oesophageal compression, gastritis, gastro-enteritis, food poisoning, dietary indiscretion (including alcohol), gastric ulcer, pyloric stenosis, gastric volvulus, duodenal ulcer, cholecystitis, pancreatitis, intestinal obstruction, appendicitis, strangulated hernia, severe constipation*
Central nervous system (CNS) disease	Raised intracranial pressure (ICP), meningitis, brain-stem stroke, Menière's disease*, labyrinthitis*
Metabolic/chemical	Drugs (especially antibiotics, opiates, chemotherapy, digoxin, oestrogens), pregnancy, diabetic ketoacidosis, uraemia, hypercalcaemia*
Reflex/constitutional	MI, any severe infection, glaucoma*

**Rare*

History

Take a careful history, including associated symptoms such as diarrhoea, abdominal pain, weight loss, headache. Do not forget to ask about drugs and alcohol. In young women, ask about the date of the last menstrual period.

Examination

This needs to include an assessment of the patient's state of hydration and a careful review of the abdomen. *Do not forget the hernial orifices.*

Investigations

Baseline tests will usually include an FBC and U & E. If there is abdominal pain, ask for a serum amylase. If there is a significant chance of a 'surgical' cause, discuss the case with your SHO or registrar; you may need to consider a plain X-ray of the abdomen (erect and supine). In young women, consider a pregnancy test.

Management

This will depend largely on the cause. It is usually possible to give an anti-emetic i.m. or i.v. such as prochlorperazine or metoclopramide. If the nausea is secondary to chemotherapy, ondansetron may be more effective. If the patient is dehydrated, rehydrate with i.v., normal saline and 5% glucose (→ p 160).

If a 'surgical' cause is likely, keep the patient nil by mouth until seen by the surgeons. If vomiting is profuse, ask the nursing staff to pass a nasogastric tube.

HAEMATEMESIS OR MELAENA

First a few basic points about haematemesis and melaena:

- Altered food in the vomitus can resemble altered blood. Do not ask the patient a leading question such as: 'Did it look like coffee grounds?' Try to be neutral when asking about the colour of vomitus and stools.
- Patients' estimates of the volume of blood lost by haematemesis are notoriously inaccurate: try to obtain more information from a witness.
- Blood mixed with the stool can arise from bleeding in *any part* of the GI tract. Similarly, melaena may occur with both upper and lower G1 tract bleeding. A history of blood per rectum (PR) is only of value for localization if the blood is bright red and liquid *and* there is no melaena *and* no haematemesis.
- If the patient is taking oral iron, the stools will be dark grey but they are usually firmer than melaena and have a different odour.

Causes (→ Tables 2.12, 2.13, 2.14)

Table 2.12 **Causes of haematemesis**
Mallory-Weiss tear Oesophagitis Gastritis (including alcoholic) Gastric erosions Gastric ulcer Duodenitis Duodenal ulcer Oesophageal varices Angiodysplasia Gastric carcinoma
Additional contributory factors Steroids NSAIDs Coagulation disorders Over-anticoagulation (warfarin, heparin, streptokinase)

Table 2.13
Causes of melaena

All of the conditions in Table 2.12, especially:

- Duodenal ulcer
- Gastric ulcer
- Oesophageal varices

Right-sided colonic lesions, e.g. angiodysplasia, carcinoma

Table 2.14
Causes of Bleeding PR

All of the conditions in Tables 2.12 and 2.13

Other colonic disorders:

- Inflammatory bowel disease
- Carcinoma
- Polyps
- Diverticular disease
- Ischaemic colitis

Anorectal conditions:

- Fissure-in-ano
- Haemorrhoids

APPROACH TO THE PATIENT WITH GI BLEEDING

- Has there been a significant bleed? If the patient has lost more than 100 ml of blood or there has been definite haematemesis or definite melaena then the bleeding is significant
- Is the patient shocked? There may be obvious signs such as pallor, cold, clammy skin, tachycardia (> 100 per min) or hypotension (systolic BP < 100 mmHg): if present, these indicate major volume depletion (several litres). If there are no obvious signs of shock you should check for postural hypotension (BP lying versus sitting upright): if the systolic BP falls by 25 mmHg or more or drops to below 100 mmHg then the patient is volume depleted.

If there is evidence of shock or volume depletion then resuscitation must be carried out immediately: detailed history and examination can be carried out during or after resuscitation.

Resuscitation in volume-depleted patients

1. Take blood for FBC, U & E, cross match (whole blood, not packed red cells; order at least 4 units initially), and clotting screen.
2. Insert the largest i.v. cannula possible.
3. Give one or two units of plasma expander (Haemaccel or Gelofusin) as rapidly as possible, then give blood as soon as it is available.
4. **Inform your SHO or registrar of the patient's existence and for assessment.** He/she should inform the surgical team on call and the on-call endoscopist. A CVP line may be needed to monitor fluid replacement.
5. Arrange admission of the patient to a high-dependency area. This is especially important if the patient is aged over 60
6. Keep the patient nil by mouth and ask the nurses to do quarter-hourly pulse and BP.
7. If the patient is aged over 40, obtain an ECG.
8. If liver disease is present, avoid sedation. Clear the bowel with magnesium sulphate mixture, 10 ml 3 times a day or an enema.
9. *Do not* give intravenous ranitidine: these are obvious theoretical attractions, but clinical trials have failed to show any benefit from such treatment in acute GI bleeding.

FURTHER ASSESSMENT

History

- Try to find out as much as you can about the circumstances of the acute bleed and about associated symptoms such as nausea, vomiting, diarrhoea or abdominal pain.
- Ask about previous history of peptic ulcer or GI haemorrhage.
- Ask about previous liver disease, heart, lung or renal diseases and about alcohol intake.
- Review the drug history, especially in relation to steroids and NSAIDs.

Examination

- If the patient is elderly or infirm or if there is a relevant history, check the cardiovascular and respiratory systems for evidence of disease.
- Examine the abdomen carefully.
- Perform a rectal examination.

FURTHER MANAGEMENT

Endoscopy

If the patient has required resuscitation then endoscopy should be performed urgently (within 12 h of admission). If the patient is less severely ill endoscopy should be performed 24–48 hours after admission. Once it is clear that endoscopy will be required you should explain the procedure to the patient and obtain signed consent.

Management of bleeding oesophageal varices

This condition constitutes a grave emergency, so *inform your seniors as early as possible.* Under no circumstances should you give drugs for variceal bleeding or try to pass a Sengstaken tube without the active involvement of a more senior person.

SWALLOWING DIFFICULTIES

Difficulty in swallowing is commonly associated with a sore throat due to an upper respiratory tract infection. If dysphagia rather than sore throat is the main symptom, however, it needs to be taken seriously as many of the causes are malignant. If the complaint is of a lump in the throat not associated with eating then the most likely cause is either a goitre or globus hystericus.

Causes (→Table 2.5)

Table 2.15
Causes of dysphagia (in order of frequency)

- Hiatus hernia
- Oesophagitis
- Brainstem stroke
- Peptic stricture secondary to long-standing reflux
- Carcinoma of the oesophagus or stomach
- Extrinsic compression (carcinoma of bronchus, lymphadenopathy, retrosternal goitre, etc.)
- Neuromuscular disorders, e.g. Guillain-Barré syndrome, Parkinson's disease, diabetic neuropathy, multiple sclerosis, myasthenia gravis, motor neurone disease, achalasia

History

As well as the dysphagia itself, you should ask about other associated symptoms such as weight loss, dyspepsia and/or reflux, hoarseness. More specifically:

- If the dysphagia is worse for solids than for liquids a mechanical obstruction is likely. If, however, the problem is as bad or worse with liquids as with solids, a motility disorder is more likely (e.g. achalasia, diabetic neuropathy).
- If it is difficult to perform the swallowing movement (and especially if the patient coughs on swallowing), bulbar or pseudobulbar palsy should come high on your list.
- If the dysphagia is constant you are probably dealing with a malignant stricture or a progressive neurological disorder.

Examination

This is often normal but it is nevertheless useful to check for the following:

- evidence of wasting
- stridor
- physical stimulation of the swallow reflex

- a 'wet' voice: food debris from the mouth falling into an unprotected airway will do this because it will remain on the vocal cords
- the nature of the cough ('bovine', etc.)
- lymphadenopathy
- a goitre or other mass in the neck
- asymmetrical chest movement
- other evidence of malignancy such as an enlarged liver or a mass in the epigastrium.

Investigations

- Routine blood tests (FBC and U&E) will usually be requested.
- A plain CXR is often helpful (for example, in showing a large shadow behind the heart in someone with a hiatus hernia).
- More specific investigations would consist of a barium swallow and/or upper GI endoscopy with biopsy.
- In a few cases oesophageal manometry (motility disorders), video-fluoroscopy or radionuclide gastric emptying studies (motility or neuromuscular disorders) will be needed.

Management

This will obviously depend on the diagnosis.

Benign peptic strictures. These can usually be treated by endoscopic dilatation. If there is associated oesophagitis this is nowadays treated with a proton pump inhibitor (omeprazole).

Extrinsic compression. This requires surgical treatment or, if the lesion is inoperable, radiotherapy.

Carcinoma of the oesophagus or stomach. These should be treated by surgical excision if this is possible. Very often, however, excision is not possible but useful palliation can be achieved either by passing a tube through the lesion or by burning away part of the tumour by means of an endoscopic laser.

Neuromuscular disorders. These require a variety of approaches.

> In cases of difficult dysphagia, especially those due to neuromuscular disorders, advice from, and involvement of, a speech therapist is often invaluable. Close liaison with a dietitian regarding nutrition is also important.

Muscular incoordination or a peripheral neuropathy. A motility agent such as domperidone or cisapride may be effective.

Bulbar or pseudobulbar palsy. The patient should be assessed by a doctor experienced in rehabilitation and by a speech therapist.

Total inability to swallow. It may be necessary to introduce a fine-bore nasogastric tube so as to provide water and nutrients. Remember that rehabilitation of the swallow can take place while nasogastric feeding is being carried out.

DIARRHOEA

Diarrhoea is defined as the passage of loose, semisolid or liquid stools, which are passed at a frequency greater than is usual for the patient.

Causes (→ Table 2.16)

Table 2.16
Causes of diarrhoea in the UK

Food poisoning/infections	*Staphylococcus aureus*, Salmonella, viruses (Norwalk, Rotavirus), *Campylobacter*, *Escherichia coli*, *Clostridium perfringens*
Inflammatory	Ulcerative colitis, Crohn's disease, pseudomembranous colitis, (patients who have been on antibiotics for several days)
Drugs	Antibiotics, laxatives, antacids, methyldopa, digoxin, colchicine
Miscellaneous	Diverticular disease, malabsorption, ischaemic colitis, colonic neoplasm, thyrotoxicosis, faecal impaction with overflow, irritable bowel syndrome

In subjects who have recently been abroad, consider tropical diseases such as amoebiasis, cholera, shigella.

History

- Ask about the timing of the diarrhoea (both onset and frequency) and about details of the stool character, i.e. whether it is completely liquid or semi-formed, the colour, whether the stool is greasy and offensive (as in malabsorption), presence of blood or mucus in the stool.
- Ask about the health of family and friends, about contact with known infectious disease and about foreign travel.
- Ask about associated symptoms such as weight loss, abdominal pain, nausea and vomiting.

Examination

- Assess state of hydration (eyes, skin turgor, fall in BP from lying to standing).
- Note whether the patient is febrile.
- Examine the abdomen and do a rectal examination.

In the elderly a rectal examination must be performed to exclude faecal impaction.

Clinical syndromes

- Antibiotic-induced: usually begins 2 or 3 days into a course of antibiotics.
- Acute food poisoning: vomiting and diarrhoea within 24 hours of ingesting contaminated food. Symptoms are caused by a bacterial toxin.
- Acute watery diarrhoea: caused by enterotoxin-producing or invasive organisms transmitted by contaminated water or food. May be caused either by viruses (Rotavirus, Norwalk) or bacteria (*E. coli, Salmonella, Vibrio cholerae*).
- Diarrhoea due to a carcinoma of colon: may be sub-acute and intermittent. Should be thought of especially in older patients or if there is blood or a lot of mucus in the stool.
- Bloody diarrhoea: blood mixed with the stool suggests a *serious intestinal infection* or the presence of *IBD*. If the stool consists entirely of fairly fresh blood, check for haemorrhoids; a bloody stool associated with abdominal pain suggests ischaemic colitis.
- Chronic diarrhoea alternating with constipation in a patient who is relatively well and has not lost weight suggests irritable bowel syndrome. Chronic diarrhoea with pale stools, weight loss and chronic abdominal pain suggests malabsorption secondary to chronic pancreatitis.

Investigations

Blood tests. These should be performed in all but mild cases; they include FBC, U&E, blood cultures (if febrile or if *Salmonella* infection is suspected), blood glucose or thyroid function tests where appropriate.

Stool examination. Send samples for culture and sensitivity. If there has been foreign travel or contact with infectious disease, send a sample for ova, cysts and parasites. If the patient is ill, dehydrated or has a high fever, immediate microscopy of a direct stool smear is indicated: the presence of polymorphs indicates that the diarrhoea is probably due to *E. coli, Campylobacter* or *Shigella*; if there are no polymorphs, *Salmonella, E. coli* or *Clostridium difficile* are likely.

X-rays. If inflammatory bowel disease is suspected, the patient must have a plain X-ray of the abdomen to look for toxic dilatation of the colon; this may need to be repeated daily.

Barium enema is sometimes necessary in patients with diarrhoea. Consult a more senior colleague.

Other tests. Sigmoidoscopy (*without* prior bowel preparation) should be carried out within the first 24 hours if IBD is suspected. Ultrasound or CT scanning of the abdomen may be indicated if a pancreatic cause is suspected. Rarely, a faecal fat collection will be required in patients suspected of having malabsorption.

Management

Isolation. Any patient suspected of having an infectious cause for diarrhoea should be isolated in a single room and barrier-nursed. Involve the control of infection nurse and his/her team.

Rehydration. This may be carried out orally in milder cases. You will need to give about 50 ml per kg initially, i.e. 2.5–3.5 litres in the first 12 hours, followed by a similar volume in each 24 hours. If the patient is anorexic, vomiting or more severely ill, rehydration should be by intravenous infusion using roughly equal parts of 0.9% saline and 5% glucose, with at least 40 mmol of potassium per litre. 4–6 litres of fluid per day may be required, depending on the severity of the diarrhoea (→ p 160–161).

> In patients needing i.v. rehydration because of diarrhoea, U&E measurements must be carried out at least once per day.

Anti-diarrhoeal drugs. These should be *avoided* in all but mild cases since, if infection is present, they will prolong it. If symptomatic anti-diarrhoeal treatment is required, use loperamide or codeine phosphate.

Antibiotics. These are not required in most cases of infective diarrhoea. If a positive stool culture is obtained or if diarrhoea persists for more than 5 days, consult your local microbiologist. As a general rule, the antibiotic agents used in infective diarrhoea are those listed in Table 2.17.

Table 2.17
Antibiotic agents used in infective diarrhoea

Organism	Antibiotic
Salmonella	Ampicillin,co-trimoxazole, chloramphenicol
Campylobacter	Erythromycin, ciprofloxacin, tetracycline
Clostridium difficile	Vancomycin, metronidazole
Yersinia	Tetracycline

Steroids and other drugs for inflammatory bowel disease. Any patient with IBD who is ill enough to need hospital admission will usually require systemic steroids, such as prednisolone 60–80 mg per day or hydrocortisone 100 mg i.v. 6 hourly. Other drugs such as rectal steroids or a 5-ASA derivative (sulphasalazine, mesalazine) may be required: consult your SHO or registrar.

JAUNDICE

Traditional teaching states that jaundice can have a haemolytic, a hepatic or an obstructive cause; however this division is of limited diagnostic value in practice.

Causes

The common causes of jaundice in adults are:

- viral hepatitis (A, B, C or D)
- alcoholic hepatitis
- biliary obstruction, due either to gallstones or to malignancy
- drug-induced jaundice (either hepatitic or cholestatic)
- multiple hepatic metastases
- cirrhosis (late stage).

Very sick patients, especially those with septicaemia, may also become jaundiced, as may patients with congestive heart failure (rarely). Jaundice in a patient who is otherwise reasonably well should make you think of inherited conditions such as Gilbert's and Crigler-Najjar syndrome.

In order to make a diagnosis, you should consider the following.

History

Ask:

- how long the patient has been jaundiced
- whether there have been pale stools or dark urine
- alcohol history in detail (including previous drinking)
- contact with infectious disease in family and friends
- foreign travel
- drug history, especially phenytoin, rifampicin, methyldopa, oral testosterone
- abdominal pain
- weight loss
- recent blood transfusion
- homosexual behaviour in men (a cause of hepatitis B)
- drug abuse.

Physical examination

Check for:

- signs of chronic liver disease, i.e. spider naevi, clubbing, Dupuytren's contracture, testicular atrophy, palmar erythema
- evidence of hepatomegaly, nodularity of the liver, pain and tenderness in the abdomen, splenomegaly, ascites.

Contrary to traditional teaching, the liver can be enlarged in a patient with cirrhosis, especially if there is associated alcoholic hepatitis or fatty infiltration. Another clinical myth is that painless jaundice is always due to malignancy. It is quite possible for obstruction secondary to gallstones to produce painless jaundice.

It is also a good idea to look for signs which will help you to assess the degree of liver dysfunction, for example the extent of any spontaneous bruising. Hepatic encephalopathy should be tested for by checking for the presence of a flapping tremor; another useful test is to ask the patient to copy a five-pointed star.

Investigations

- Test the urine (by dipstix) for urobilinogen (which indicates haemolysis) and for bilirubin (found in hepatitis and obstruction).
- Send off blood for LFTs, hepatitis A, B and C serology, full blood count and coagulation screen. The LFTs will often give valuable clues as to the cause of the jaundice (Fig. 2.1).

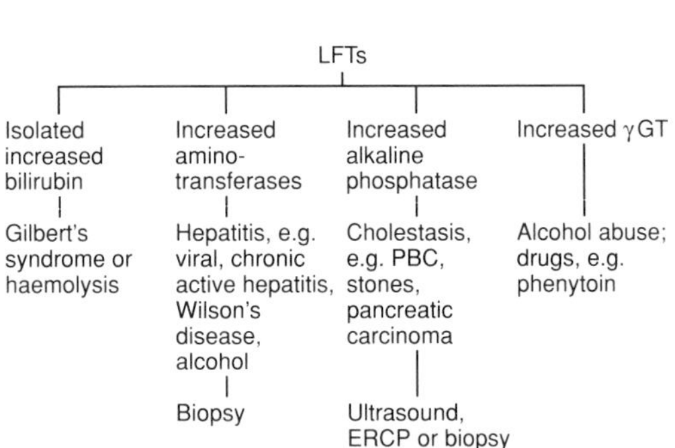

Fig 2.1
Scheme for the differential diagnosis of jaundice.

Patients with jaundice should *always* be assumed to represent a high risk for transmission of hepatitis and all specimens from these patients should be labelled as 'high risk'.

- If there is a possibility of obstruction, cirrhosis or metastases, ask for an ultrasound scan of the liver.
- If there is a possibility of autoimmune disease or chronic liver disease, send blood for anti-nuclear factor and antibodies against smooth muscle and mitochondria.
- If you are considering haemolysis, ask for haptoglobin, a blood film and a Coombs' test.

Management

Treatment of the jaundiced patient will obviously depend on the cause. The patient should be carefully observed for evidence of hepatic decompensation and encephalopathy, with regular checks on clotting status and blood count. If there is evidence of decompensation, treatment should include:

- a high carbohydrate, low protein, very low salt diet
- large doses of thiamine
- intravenous vitamin K if there is a clotting abnormality
- regular culture of blood, urine, etc. and aggressive treatment of any infection
- oral lactulose and neomycin
- avoidance of sedatives.

LIVER ENLARGEMENT

Enlargement of the liver might be found in the course of examining a patient where you are already expecting such a finding (for example a patient with alcoholic liver disease or advanced malignancy) or it may be a chance observation.

Causes (→ Table 2.18)

Table 2.18
Causes of palpable liver

Common	Alcoholic liver disease (± fatty infiltration), displacement by over-inflated lungs (asthma/chronic bronchitis), metastases, congestive cardiac failure, bile duct obstruction
Less common	Lymphoma, myelofibrosis, tricuspid incompetence, viral hepatitis (including infectious mononucleosis), primary hepatoma
Rare	Chronic liver disease not due to alcohol, polycystic liver, constrictive pericarditis, carcinoid syndrome, Riedel's lobe, Budd-Chiari syndrome, haemolytic anaemia, infiltrations (amyloid, sarcoid,etc.)

A patient with cirrhosis may have an enlarged liver. It is only in advanced cirrhosis that the liver becomes small and shrunken.

UNSUSPECTED LIVER ENLARGEMENT

History
Review the history, asking about:

- alcohol intake
- previous history of liver disease
- previous history of heart disease
- weight loss
- contact with infectious disease.

Examination

- General examination: look for evidence of chronic liver disease (jaundice, palmar erythema, spider naevi, Dupuytren's contracture).
- Check for enlarged lymph nodes.

- Examine the heart and chest, looking for evidence of heart failure, hyper-inflation of the lungs, abnormal or asymmetrical chest movement.
- Re-check the abdomen and try to answer the following questions:
  - Is the liver: smooth or nodular?
    tender or non-tender?
    pulsatile?
  - Is the spleen enlarged?
  - Is there ascites?
  - Are there any other abdominal masses?

Investigations

- Basic blood tests: blood count, LFTs, clotting screen, hepatitis, A, B and C.
- Further blood tests: anti-nuclear factor, auto-antibodies, glandular fever screening test (Paul-Bunnell, Monospot), alpha-foetoprotein (if hepatoma is suspected).
- Where indicated: CXR, liver ultrasound or CT scan, liver biopsy.

ASCITES

Causes (→ Table 2.19)

Table 2.19
Causes of ascites

Common	Cirrhosis, congestive heart failure, malignancy
Less Common	Nephrotic syndrome, hypoproteinaemia, abdominal trauma
Rare	Tuberculosis, constrictive pericarditis, Budd-Chiari syndrome

APPROACH

You should ask yourself:

- Is it ascites? Be sure to differentiate the swelling from other causes of abdominal distension such as fat, faeces or a mass. *Careful percussion is needed.*
- Are there any abdominal masses (including the liver and spleen)?

PARACENTESIS

This may be performed either for diagnostic purposes or to relieve symptoms (pain from severe distension, or breathlessness).

Equipment

- Minor dressing pack
- Antiseptic
- Lignocaine
- 20 ml syringe and 21-gauge needle (green) for a diagnostic tap
- For a therapeutic tap, a 60 ml Luer-lock syringe, 3-way tap, 18–G cannula (Venflon, etc.), drainage tube and a 2-litre measuring jug to act as receiver (or one-piece drain and collecting bag if the ascites is to be drained slowly). Specimen bottles for biochemistry (protein content), microbiology and cytology.

Procedure

1. Ask the patient to lie supine, as flat as is comfortably possible.
2. Percuss carefully and locate the site of maximum dullness. Clean the skin over this area with antiseptic.

3. Infiltrate the skin and subcutaneous tissues with lignocaine.
4. For a diagnostic tap, pass the needle through the abdominal wall, aspirating gently as you do so. Withdraw about 20 ml of fluid and note the colour. Remove the needle and put a dressing over the wound. Put the specimens into the respective bottles.

> Diagnostic aspirations should be done reasonably early in the day: fluid for cytology must be processed within a short time as the cells will degenerate if the specimen is kept in the fridge overnight.

5. For a therapeutic drainage, avoid the lower central abdomen where the inferior epigastric vessels lie. Attach the cannula and 3-way tap to the syringe and introduce the needle with gentle aspiration. Once fluid is flowing freely, remove the needle, leaving the cannula in place. Attach the 3-way tap and syringe to the cannula and the drainage tube to the side arm of the 3-way tap. Ask an assistant to hold the receiver under the drainage tube. Aspirate until the fluid ceases to flow freely or until you have withdrawn 1.5 litres. Remember to send specimens for protein, culture and cytology. If you are leaving a drain in situ, this can be introduced using an enclosed needle or with a trochar. If you are not sure how to use this, consult someone more senior.

RENAL IMPAIRMENT OR A POOR URINE OUTPUT

PATIENTS AT RISK

A poor urine output and/or renal function is particularly likely in association with:

- pre-existing renal disease
- widespread atherosclerosis
- diabetes
- dehydration
- hypotension or a poor cardiac output
- nephrotoxic drugs such as gentamicin, gold, penicillamine, cytotoxic drugs, paracetamol, tetracyclines
- septicaemia and DIC
- bladder or pelvic tumours (including prostate).

The problem will usually declare itself in the form of a rising urea or creatinine or an evident fall-off in urine output. A healthy person should pass more than 30 ml urine/hour. Sometimes it may be noticed because of progressive symptoms (drowsiness, apathy, anorexia, nausea, oedema). When faced with a patient whose urine output/renal function are deteriorating, the normal diagnostic process is reversed, as the priorities are:

- to assess the causes and treatment of the *immediate* deterioration
- to consider underlying causes of renal impairment.

MANAGEMENT

The immediate management of the situation is summarized in Table 2.20.

Table 2.20
Management of renal impairment or poor urine output

Question	Action
Is the patient dehydrated?	• Assess skin turgor, venous pressure and BP, lying and standing: if the systolic pressure falls by more than 25 mm or falls below 100 mm when the patient stands up, this is good evidence of volume depletion • If the patient is dehydrated and there is no risk of provoking pulmonary oedema it is reasonable to give a fluid challenge in the form of 500 ml normal saline • If there is postural hypotension, give a unit of plasma expander (Haemaccel, Gelofusin) • Look for other treatable causes of hypotension (→ pp 50 – 54) • If blood loss has occurred (remember to check drains if the patient has had a recent operation) replace with whole blood (not packed cells)
Is there outflow obstruction?	• Examine the abdomen to see if the bladder is distended • Perform a rectal examination • Catheterize the patient so that urine flow can be measured; if the patient is already catheterized ask the nursing staff to wash the catheter out to check that it is not blocked

Table 2.20 (cont.)

	• Ask for a plain KUB X-ray to look for stones • Consider an ultrasound scan to look for evidence of obstruction
Is the patient receiving any nephrotoxic drugs?	• Review admission drug history and the current prescription sheet
Is the patient septicaemic ?	• Briefly review history and examination. Take blood for culture if pyrexial • Check coagulation screen, platelet count and fibrinogen titre (or D-dimer)
Is the patient hyperkalaemic?	• If serum potassium is greater than 5.5 mmol, give calcium resonium by mouth or by enema • If greater than 6.5 mmol, attach a cardiac monitor • If there are ECG changes (bradycardia; tall, peaked T waves, widened QRS complexes), give 10 ml of 10% calcium gluconate i.v. immediately • For all patients with serum $K^+ > 6.5$, whether ECG is abnormal or not, give i.v. injection of 50 g of glucose plus 15 units of soluble insulin. Then *inform your SHO or registrar*
Is there any evidence of underlying renal disease or nephropathic illness?	• Ask about previous kidney diseases, haematuria, hypertension • Consider myeloma in the elderly • Consider hypercalcaemia, especially in patients with malignancy

FURTHER MANAGEMENT

The further management of renal failure should be discussed with a more senior member of the firm. It is likely to involve some or all of the following:

- intravenous fluids (see 'renal cocktail')
- oral or intravenous diuretics
- control of infection
- careful monitoring of fluid balance, serum electrolytes, body weight and CVP
- dopamine infusion to assist renal blood flow (N.B. this drug **must never** be given via a peripheral vein)
- inotropic support in the case of hypotension
- peritoneal dialysis or haemodialysis.

You may also need to consider further investigations such as ultrasound scan, serum protein electrophoresis, urinary protein measurement, urine osmolality, urinary U&E.

Fluid replacement in renal failure

If the patient is oliguric (less than 500 ml per 24 h), the patient should be rehydrated if necessary, then given a total of 500 ml per 24 hours plus the previous day's output. This should be given as 5% or 10% glucose.

If there is any doubt about the hydration status of a patient with renal failure, the CVP should be measured.

If the patient is not oliguric but has a high urea and creatinine then a 'renal cocktail' may be given consisting of three fluids in rotation:

- 500 ml of 10% glucose
- 500 ml of normal saline
- 500 ml of 1.26% sodium bicarbonate.

The fluid should be infused at 80 ml/hour. Potassium may be added if required. Watch carefully for overhydration.

Urinary catheterization (→ p135)

ACUTE PAIN IN THE LEG

This section is concerned with pain which affects the whole of the calf or the whole leg, not pain confined to a single joint or a pair of joints.

Causes (→ Table 2.21)

Table 2.21 Causes of acute pain in the leg
Mechanical: trauma, sprain, etc
Thrombophlebitis
DVT
Cellulitis
Ruptured knee joint/ruptured Baker's cyst
Embolism to the femoral artery or its branches
Neuropathic pain, e.g. diabetes

History

Ask about:

- duration of the pain
- nature of the pain
- whether it came on gradually or suddenly
- whether it affects the whole leg or a part
- whether it is worse when walking or when the patient moves to stand up
- any history of previous DVT
- in women, ask about the oral contraceptive pill.

Examination

1. Inspect the leg for:
   - skin colour
   - temperature (use the back of your hand)
   - swelling
   - distended veins
   - breaks in skin, blisters, ulcers, etc.
2. If you think the leg is swollen, measure the circumference with a tape measure. For the calf, identify the tibial tuberosity on each side, then measure 10 cm down from this on the anterior surface. Mark the skin with a pen and measure the circumference just below the mark. A difference of 2 cm or more between the two sides is significant. For the thigh, measure 25 cm from the anterior superior iliac spine and mark the leg with a pen. A difference of 2 cm or more between the two sides is significant.
3. Check for the presence of femoral, popliteal and foot pulses.
4. If you think the pain might be neuropathic, check light

touch, pinprick and vibration sense (joint position sense is not helpful in this situation) and examine the knee and ankle reflexes.

Clinical syndromes

Deep vein thrombosis (DVT). The history is usually of a fairly rapid (but not abrupt) onset of pain, over a period of hours. The patient may say that he or she has been immobile for some time prior to the event (e.g. a long coach or plane journey). There may be a history of recent use of oral contraceptives. The pain may get acutely worse if the patient puts the foot to the ground to stand up. On examination the affected leg is swollen, warm and pink and there may be visible distended veins. The calf may be acutely tender posteriorly and Homan's sign may be positive (pain in the posterior calf on dorsiflexion of the foot) but the lack of a positive Homan's sign should not put you off the diagnosis of DVT.

Cellulitis. There may be a history of recent bite or trauma to the leg. On examination, the affected area is hot, swollen and red (the redness is usually much more marked than in DVT). The affected area of the leg may have an irregular boundary which does not follow obvious anatomical landmarks.

Ruptured knee joint/Baker's cyst. There may be a history of arthritis (either osteo or rheumatoid) in the relevant knee. On examination the leg is swollen and may be very red and tender over the posterior and lateral calf.

> **Venous thrombosis is rare in rheumatoid arthritis. If a patient with known rheumatoid arthritis develops a painful, swollen calf it is much more likely to be a ruptured knee joint than a DVT.**

Arterial thromboembolism. The pain comes on very abruptly and is often intense. There may be a previous history of atherosclerotic vascular disease, valvular heart disease or atrial fibrillation. The leg is often very pale, sometimes with peripheral purplish or bluish discoloration, and feels cold.

> **The acutely ischaemic leg is a surgical emergency : contact your SHO or a member of the on-call vascular surgical team immediately (see below).**

Neuropathic pain. This is characteristically sharp and stabbing or burning in nature, or the patient may say that it feels like walking on sharp pebbles. On examination there is usually impairment of at least one sensory modality and absence of the ankle jerks.

Investigations

- If there are any broken areas of skin or ulcers, take swabs from these for culture.
- If the patient is febrile or you suspect cellulitis, take blood cultures.
- If you suspect a DVT, even if you are not sure, the patient *must* have a venogram as the diagnosis can be extremely difficult to make clinically. If there is going to be any delay in obtaining a venogram the patient should be given analgesics and i.v. heparin (→ below and p 208); remember to check a coagulation screen before starting heparin.
- If you suspect a ruptured knee joint the investigation of choice will be an arthrogram; it is wise to discuss the case with your SHO or registrar before ordering this.

Management

Deep venous thrombosis (DVT). The patient should be given analgesia and commenced on i.v. heparin: give a bolus dose of 5000 u and follow this with an infusion of 1400 u per hour via an infusion pump. After about 10 hours, check the APTT and adjust the heparin infusion rate as necessary (→ p 209). Once the diagnosis of DVT is confirmed, start treatment with warfarin, 10 mg in the early evening; adjust the dose as indicated in Table 4.6 (p 212). Once the patient has had heparin for 5 days *and* the INR is within the therapeutic range, the heparin can be stopped. Warfarin will need to be continued for 3–6 months (each consultant will have a special preference).

The patient should be fitted with an elastic, graduated compression stocking (T.E.D. stocking) and early mobilization encouraged.

If the patient has had a large ilio-femoral thrombosis and there is a lot of tension in the tissues, there is a risk of venous gangrene and streptokinase may be needed: consult your SHO or registrar.

Cellulitis. Give analgesics and antibiotics in the form of benzylpenicillin, 600 mg 6 hourly i.v. plus flucloxacillin, 250 mg 6 hourly i.v. If penicillin-allergic, give erythromycin, 1 gm 6 hourly i.v. The leg should be supported on a footstool or on pillows.

Arterial embolism. This constitutes a surgical *emergency*: either you or your SHO/registrar should contact the on-call vascular surgical team immediately. The patient may well need to go to theatre, so check that he/she has had a recent FBC, U & E and ECG and take blood for group and save. Begin anticoagulation with i.v. heparin, 5000 u as a bolus injection, followed by 1400 u per hour.

Ruptured knee joint. Initially (before the diagnosis is proven) give analgesics, which may be continued as needed after the arthrogram. If you think that someone may have had either a

DVT or a ruptured knee joint, remember that heparin is *contraindicated* in cases of ruptured joint. The treatment is analgesics and rest initially, followed by mobilization with a supportive elastic stocking.

EXCESSIVE BRUISING OR BLEEDING

Causes (→ Table 2.22)

Table 2.22
Causes of excessive bruising or bleeding
(Causes in order of frequency)

Diagnosis	Causes
Connective tissue atrophy	Old age Steroid therapy Wasting
Thrombocytopaenia	Viral infections Drug induced (inc. alcohol) B_{12} or folate deficiency bone marrow dyscrasias ↑ consumption (idiopathic thrombocytopenic purpura (ITP), DIC, hypersplenism) Systemic lupus erythematosus (SLE)
Clotting factor deficiency	Liver disease Drug induced (heparin, warfarin) Excess consumption (DIC) Dilution (large blood transfusion) Congenital (haemophilia, etc.) Vitamin K deficiency (e.g. malabsorption)
Vessel wall disorders	Aspirin Osler-Weber-Rendu disease Angiodysplasia

History

The most important questions relating to the haemorrhagic disorder are:

- Has this ever happened before?
- Have you lost weight?
- Have you been feverish or otherwise generally unwell?
- What drugs or medicines have you had recently (a full, detailed drug history, including over-the-counter medications, is essential → Table 2.23)?

- How much alcohol do you drink?
- Is there a family history of any similar problem?

Table 2.23
Drugs causing thrombocytopaenia

Cytotoxic therapy
Diuretics (thiazides, frusemide)
NSAIDs (including aspirin)
Sulphonamides
Rifampicin
Quinidine
Methyldopa
Penicillins
Lots of others

Examination

Look especially for:

- evidence of anaemia
- bruising or bleeding inside the mouth
- the pattern of bruising in the skin
- lymph node enlargement
- signs of chronic liver disease (spider naevi, palmar erythema, Dupuytren's contracture, oedema, ascites, splenomegaly, testicular atrophy)
- enlargement of the liver or spleen.

It is also wise to examine the eyes for signs of fundal haemorrhage as this has important implications for the management of the patient.

Clinical patterns. Below are a few observations which may give you a clue as to the cause of the bleeding disorder.

- Purpura is common in platelet disorders but rare in diseases affecting clotting factors.
- In platelet disorders bruising is usually multiple and superficial, while in coagulopathies it is deeper and often single.
- Vascular and platelet disorders lead to prolonged bleeding from superficial cuts, whereas clotting factor abnormalities produce delayed bleeding from deeper structures such as muscles, joints, gastrointestinal tract (GIT).
- Bleeding from mucous membranes is usually due to a platelet or blood vessel disorder.
- Bleeding from needle puncture sites should make you think of DIC.

Investigations

- FBC, platelet count and blood film.
- PT and KCCT (APTT).

- If DIC is suspected (→ Table 2.24), ask for a fibrinogen titre and/or a measure of fibrin degradation products such as D-dimer; your local haematology laboratory will advise you if you are unsure.
- **Remember to take blood for group and cross-match.**

Table 2.24 **Causes of DIC**
Septicaemia, especially Gram-negative or meningococcal
Obstetric causes
intrauterine death
abruptio placentae
amniotic fluid embolism
Incompatible blood transfusion
Pancreatitis
Anaphylaxis
Malignancy, especially promyelocytic leukaemia
Major surgery, especially with extra-corporeal shunts

Laboratory features of DIC include the following:

- reduced platelet count
- prolonged PT, KCCT and thrombin time
- reduced fibrinogen titre
- increased fibrin degradation products (or D-dimer)
- fragmented red cells on blood film.

Management

You will almost certainly want to involve your SHO/registrar in the patient's management. However, a few basic principles can be stated.

- **i.m injections are absolutely contraindicated** in someone with a clotting disorder: it is best to write, in red, on the drug prescription sheet: 'No i.m. injections'. By the same token, invasive vascular procedures such as CVP line insertion, should be undertaken with great caution, if at all, in patients with clotting defects (and should *not* be undertaken by you).
- Transfused platelets are rapidly consumed and repeated transfusion can give rise to platelet antibodies which would make subsequent transfusion of platelets impossible. Platelet transfusion should not, therefore, be undertaken on the basis of the count alone unless this is very low (less than 25 x 10^9). The indications for platelet transfusion are related to active bleeding, as judged by:
  - externally visible bleeding (GIT, etc.)
  - new bleeding into the skin (petechiae or purpura)
  - CNS bleeding (including fundal haemorrhage)
  - cover for intercurrent surgery.

It is vital, therefore, to examine the skin and the optic fundi *daily* in any patient with moderate or severe thrombocytopenia.

- If the patient has a deficiency of clotting factors (liver disease, overtreatment with warfarin, DIC, etc.) and is actively bleeding, FFP should be given in order to replace them. A cross-match will need to be performed before FFP is given. It is usually administered in a dose of two units or four units at a time (run in fairly quickly). If the patient is volume depleted or is actively bleeding, fresh blood should be given. The coagulation defect may be corrected by giving the patient vitamin K as phytomenadione, 5 mg *intravenously*, given slowly.
- Patients with haemophilia who present with an acute bleed will require cryoprecipitate or factor VIII concentrate. Consult your local haematologist.

UNCONSCIOUSNESS AND DEPRESSED CONSCIOUS LEVEL

To be presented with a patient who is unconscious without known cause is a very stressful experience. If the patient has severe or total depression of consciousness you should, **before doing anything** else:

- Make sure that you are not dealing with a cardiac arrest, i.e. check that the patient has a palpable carotid or femoral pulse.
- Note whether the patient is cyanosed or appears to have an abnormal breathing pattern (for example, Cheyne-Stokes breathing). Check that the airway is clear.
- Check the BP.

> ⚠ **If the patient's immediate survival seems in danger, call for help from your SHO or registrar.**

CAUSES OF DEPRESSED CONSCIOUSNESS

Transient loss/depression of consciousness

(→ Table 2.25)

Table 2.25
Causes of transient depression of conciousness

Most common	Stroke/TIA, cardiac arrhythmia, MI
Common	Epileptic fit,simple faint, head injury, hypoglycaemia,cardiomyopathy
Uncommon	Aortic stenosis, Subdural haematoma

Sustained loss of consciousness (→ Table 2.26)

Table 2.26
Causes of sustained depression of consciousness

Most common	Stroke/TIA, sub-arachnoid haemorrhage, head injury, drug overdose (including alcohol), cardiogenic shock, cardiac arrhythmia, epilepsy
Common	meningitis, poisoning (e.g. carbon monoxide, respiratory failure, renal failure, hepatic failure, shock 2^0 to blood loss, hypoglycaemia, hyperglycaemia ± ketoacidosis, encephalitis, hypothermia, subdural haematoma
Uncommon	Hypothyroidism, psychosis hypercalcaemia

HISTORY

This will usually be obtained from witnesses rather than the patient. The speed of onset is of prime importance. Hepatic failure, for example, does not come on suddenly without any foregoing illness. Ask about previous diseases (e.g. diabetes) and recent symptoms such as:

- fever
- headache
- unsteadiness
- weakness on one side
- mental clouding
- slurring of speech
- chest pain
- breathlessness
- haematemesis and melaena.

EXAMINATION

Assess the patient's level of consciousness in terms of the Glasgow coma scale (GCS) (→ Table 2.27).

Table 2.27
Glasgow coma scale

Score	*Motor response*	*Verbal response*	*Eye opening*
6	Obeys simple commands	–	–
5	Attempts to remove source of painful stimuli to head or trunk	Orientated	–
4	Attempts to withdraw from source of pain	Disorientated	Eyes open
3	Flexes arm at elbow and wrist in response to nail-bed pressure	Random speech	Open to speech
2	Extends arms at elbow and wrist in response to nail-bed pressure	Mumbling	Open to pain
1	No motor response to painful stimuli	No speech	No opening

Add the individual scores to obtain the final total. Best = 15, worst = 3.

Examine each system in turn, looking especially for:

- brady- or tachycardia
- BP
- cardiac murmurs
- abnormal respiratory pattern
- signs of peritonitis
- signs of aortic aneurysm
- signs of GI bleeding (a rectal examination is essential)
- meningism
- papilloedema
- facial asymmetry or asymmetry of limb posture
- reflexes.

INVESTIGATIONS

Transient loss of consciousness

Investigations will be guided by the history and examination. A blood glucose is useful in most cases. If the patient is over 40 or there is any reason to suspect an arrhythmia, an ECG should be performed.

Sustained loss of consciousness

All patients should have:

- blood count
- U&E
- blood glucose
- ECG.

If the clinical features are suggestive, you may need to arrange:

- blood gas estimation
- drug levels
- CXR.

In the case of head injury or suspected meningitis or subarachnoid haemorrhage, a CT brain scan is often necessary. Consult your SHO or registrar.

> **In a patient with focal neurological signs or where there is a suspicion of raised ICP, lumbar puncture must not be performed until a CT scan has been done. Absence of papilloedema does *not* mean that it is safe to do an LP. In a seriously ill patient with suspected meningitis, high dose i.v. benzyl penicillin may be given before CT scan and LP.**

MANAGEMENT

Transient loss of consciousness

This will depend on the cause.

Sustained loss of consciousness

Initial management must include securing the airway, usually by nursing the patient in the three-quarter prone position and by using a plastic airway where necessary. Make sure that the patient has an adequate BP and is well oxygenated. Urinary catheterization is often desirable in order to monitor urine output. Further treatment will depend on the cause of the condition.

HEADACHE

Causes (→ Table 2.28)

Table 2.28
Causes of headache

Common	Tension headache — A . Trauma Migraine — A Sub-arachnoid haemorrhage — A Raised ICP Meningitis — A Encephalitis — A Temporal arteritis — A
Uncommon	Hypercapnia Stroke — A Carbon monoxide poisoning Hypertensive encephalopathy Acute glaucoma — A Sinusitis Trigeminal neuralgia — A

History

Ask about:

- The onset of the headache. Those marked A above come on relatively acutely, whereas the other disorders cause chronic headache. Tension headaches can be acute or chronic.
- Site. Migraine headache is, by definition, unilateral at its onset, though it may become bilateral later. Occipital headache coming on suddenly must raise the suspicion of sub-arachnoid haemorrhage or meningitis, *even if there is no definite meningism on examination.*
- Previous history of headaches or migraine.
- Associated symptoms, e.g. nausea, photophobia, disorientation.

Examination

1. Assess the patient's level of consciousness and orientation (GCS, → p 102). If there is depression of consciousness or disorientation, you are obviously dealing with a serious cause of headache such as meningitis, encephalitis, sub-arachnoid haemorrhage, poisoning, trauma or raised ICP.
2. Check the patient's temperature, pulse and BP.
3. Look for evidence of trauma to the head.

4. Examine the eyes for signs of glaucoma (red eye, oval pupil).
5. Check for a rash (meningitis).
6. Temporal arteritis is a disease of the over-60s: in this age group, check to see whether the temporal arteries are palpable and tender.
7. Perform a quick neurological examination, checking especially for signs of meningism, that the pupils are equal and reactive, that there is no papilloedema and that there is no obvious hemiparesis. Note that hypercapnia may cause papilloedema.

It is useful to look for papilloedema, but its absence does *not* mean that raised ICP can be excluded.

In sub-arachnoid haemorrhage, you may see sub-hyaloid haemorrhages. In malignant hypertension there may be exudates or haemorrhages in the fundi.

Investigations and management

- If you suspect temporal arteritis, ask for a blood count and ESR — this need not be obtained as an emergency. Temporal artery biopsy, which can be performed after treatment has started, may be needed later. Treat suspected temporal arteritis with prednisolone, beginning with a dose of 60 mg per day. If the diagnosis of temporal arteritis is correct, the response to steroids is usually dramatic within 24–48 hours.
- If meningitis or sub-arachnoid haemorrhage is suspected, a decision needs to be made (not by you) as to whether lumbar puncture (LP) or urgent CT scanning is indicated: blind LP is not acceptable nowadays, so consult your SHO or registrar. If sub-arachnoid haemorrhage is a serious possibility, give nimodipine orally or (if the patient cannot swallow) intravenously. Give analgesia in the form of dihydrocodeine or pethidine and anti-emetics (metoclopramide or prochlorperazine). If a CT scan is thought unnecessary or has been done and is negative, LP should be performed to look for evidence of meningitis or encephalitis (→ p 138). Send cerebrospinal fluid (CSF) samples for microscopy and culture, protein and glucose and remember to send a blood sample for glucose at the same time (→ Table 2.29).

Table 2.29
CSF values in menigitis

	Normal	Bacterial	Viral	TB
Appearance:	Clear	Turbid	Clear or turbid	Turbid (may be fibrinous)
Polymorphs (per cu mm):	0	>200	<100	<100
Mononuclear cells (per cu mm):	0	<100	10–1000	100–300
Protein (gm/l):	<0.5 g/l	>1 g/l	0.5–1 g/l	1–5 g/l
Glucose:	2/3 of blood glucose	<50% of blood glucose	2/3 of blood glucose	<1/3 of blood glucose

If meningitis is suspected clinically, antibiotics must be started immediately. Do not wait for the CSF results. In adults, give i.v. benzylpenicillin, 2.4 g every 4 hours; if the patient is allergic to penicillin, give chloramphenicol, 12.5 mg per kg every 6 hours. If TB meningitis is suspected, consult a senior colleague or your local microbiologist.

If a patient has meningitis due to either *Haemophilus influenzae* or meningococcus, family and close friends should be offered prophylaxis, usually with rifampicin. Remember also that meningitis is a notifiable disease.

- Migraine should in the first instance be treated with simple analgesics (aspirin or paracetamol) and anti-emetics; ergotamine derivatives are not usually necessary. In severe cases, consider sumatriptan.
- Investigate and treat other types of headache according to their cause.

Except in cases of trauma, a skull X-ray is usually unhelpful in making a diagnosis of the cause of headache.

FITS

1. The first priority here is to make sure that the patient is 'safe' when you arrive, i.e. that the fit has stopped, the patient has a clear airway and a normal pulse rate and BP.

> **If the patient is not 'safe' when you arrive, you should bleep your SHO or registrar urgently.**

If you arrive during the fit, do not restrain the patient at all; simply wait for the fit to end and protect the patient from injury. If possible, put on a face mask and give 100% oxygen. If the fit is continuing, give diazemuls, 10–20 mg intravenously *slowly* (5 mg per min) or 10 mg rectally.

2. Try to establish from witnesses the exact nature of the attack:
   - Did the patient actually convulse?
   - Did the attack begin focally or with generalized rigidity?
   - Did the patient appear to lose consciousness?
   - Was the patient aware of any aura or behave oddly or cry out just before the attack?

> A typical *grand mal* or generalized fit begins with a tonic phase, with rigidity of the whole body, followed by convulsive jerking of the limbs and trunk. During the attack the patient may become pale or cyanosed. Afterwards the patient will often be drowsy for several minutes and there may be a short-lived focal weakness (Todd's paresis).

3. Find out if there is a past history of epilepsy.
4. Once the fit has stopped, check the patient's state of consciousness (GCS, → p 102) and carry out a quick neurological review: check especially for meningism, that the pupils are equal and reactive, that there is no papilloedema and that there is no obvious hemiparesis. If the patient is not fully conscious, nurse in the recovery position
5. Consider secondary causes of fitting (→ Table 2.30).

Table 2.30 Secondary causes of fitting	
Metabolic	Hypoglycaemia* Hypocalcaemia Hypoxia* Water intoxication Hypo- or hypernatraemia Liver failure*
Structural	Head injury* Stroke* Intracranial mass*
Infective	Encephalitis
Toxic	Phenothiazines Tricyclic antidepressants Withdrawal of alcohol or benzodiazepines*

* The most common cause

INVESTIGATIONS

In someone who has an unexpected fit with no definite cause it is wise to check the blood glucose at the bedside using a test strip (BM stix, Glucostix, etc.) and also to send blood to the laboratory for urgent U & E, glucose and blood count. If there is any suggestion of hypoxia or if the patient is having fits in quick succession, check blood gases and give 100% oxygen by face mask.

MANAGEMENT

To terminate a seizure

It is often best to wait for a few moments and simply allow the fit to subside (→ above). If, however, the fit is continuing, give diazemuls, 10–20 mg intravenously *slowly* (5 mg per min) or diazepam, 10 mg rectally.

Hypoglycaemia

If the bedside glucose test suggests hypoglycaemia, give 50 ml of 50% glucose into a large vein; if venous access is difficult, give 1 mg glucagon intramuscularly. You may need to follow this up with a glucose infusion. Consult your SHO or registrar.

Alcohol withdrawal and liver disease

Give intravenous thiamine (as Parentrovite), followed by an infusion of 10% glucose, 50 ml per hour. Regular blood glucose monitoring (2–4 hourly by a bedside method) is advisable.

Seizures without known cause

Nurse the patient in the recovery position and ensure that oxygenation and BP are adequate. Ask the nursing staff to do regular observations ('neuro. obs.') every half hour or every hour.

Recurrent fits

You should not give more than two bolus doses of diazemuls. If fitting recurs after two doses, then prepare a phenytoin infusion by diluting 250 mg of phenytoin solution in 250 ml of normal saline; give a dose of 15 mg per kg at a rate of not more than 50 mg/min (→ Table 2.31).

Table 2.31
Phenytoin dosage

Body weight, kg	Volume of phenytoin solution needed to give 15 mg/kg, ml
40	600
45	675
50	750
55	825
60	900
65	975
70	1050
75	1125
80	1200
85	1275
90	1350
95	1425
100	1500

CONFUSION

The term 'confused' has no precise definition and ideally ought not to be used at all. Patients who are described as confused often display one or more of the following features:

- disorientation, especially in place and time
- restlessness and agitation
- inability to respond appropriately to verbal requests or instructions
- incoherent, rambling or nonsensical speech
- inappropriate or bizarre behaviour.

There may also be clouding of consciousness, drowsiness, apathy or withdrawal from normal ward behaviour such as eating meals.

If you are asked to see a patient who is 'confused' try to establish exactly what the abnormal behaviour pattern is. Wherever possible, find out about the patient's normal mental state by interviewing a relative or friend. Talk to the patient yourself. Try to get an impression of how lucid or otherwise the patient is and make sure that the conversational disorder (if there is one) is not simply dysphasia. Examine the patient, checking especially:

- Temperature, pulse and BP.
- Cyanosis or respiratory distress.
- Signs in the chest. Is there evidence of a bronchopneumonia?
- Rapid neurological review: there is no need to go into minutiae but you should at least make sure that there is no meningism, that the pupils are equal and reactive, that there is no papilloedema and that there is no obvious hemiparesis.

Check that a ward urine dipstick test has been done (UTI can cause mental impairment in the elderly). Review the drug prescription sheet, looking especially for hypnotics and sedatives, antidepressants, potent analgesics. Depending on the history and examination you may need to arrange investigations such as white cell count, blood gases, blood glucose (remember alcoholism, liver disease and paracetamol poisoning as causes of hypoglycaemia), serum calcium, CXR, blood or urine cultures, U & E.

If the patient is drowsy or semi-conscious the diagnostic possibilities become more numerous (→ p 101).

MANAGEMENT

If a patient is restless or agitated and you have not found an immediately treatable cause such as hypoxia or hypoglycaemia you may need to sedate the patient. In such a case, consider:

- haloperidol, 5 mg i.m, repeated hourly if needed
- chlorpromazine, 25–50 mg i.m
- diazepam rectally
- chlormethiazole by i.v. infusion.

Cot sides are best avoided as patients may climb over them and then fall. It is better to nurse a very restless patient on a mattress on the floor in a side room. If the patient needs to continue receiving an i.v. infusion, strap this well on to the arm and bandage the arm securely. A mitten on the patient's other hand may be useful.

If the patient's mental state and/or conscious level fluctuate for no apparent reason, consider a CT scan or isotope brain scan to look for a subdural haematoma.

If you are in any doubt about the wisdom of giving sedation to the patient, consult a more senior colleague.

Table 2.32
Mini mental state examination*

1. Orientation
Ask the following questions (one point for each correct answer):

- What date is it today?
- What day of the week is it?
- Which month are we in?
- What year is it?
- Can you tell me what season it is? (Be flexible: 'spring' or 'summer' would be acceptable in June, 'autumn' or 'winter' in December, etc.)
- Can you tell me the name of the hospital?
- Which floor are we on?
- What town or city are we in?
- Which county are we in? (Or, in a town or city known to the patient, can you name a main street nearby?)
- Which country are we in?

2. Immediate recall
Ask permission to test the patient's memory. Say 'I am going to name three objects. After I have finished giving you the names I will want you to repeat them. Try and remember what they are because I shall ask you about them again later.' Then name the objects, speaking slowly and clearly (e.g. table, flag, tree). Score the patient's first try (one point for each object) but keep repeating them until the patient can say them all correctly (up to six attempts).

3. Attention and calculation
Say: 'I would like you to take away 7 from 100, then take away 7 again, and keep going.' Score one point for each correct subtraction of 7 (even if one of the answers is wrong along the way) up to the maximun of five points.

Table 2.32 (cont.)

Patients who cannot or will not attempt serial subtractions, should be asked to spell the word 'world' backward. Score one point for each letter in the correct position.

4. Recall
Ask the patient to repeat the names of the three objects given earlier; score one point for each correct answer.

5. Naming
Show a pencil or pen and ask what it is called, then do the same with a wristwatch. Score one point for each correct answer.

6. Repetition
Say (once only): 'I am going to say something and I would like you to repeat it after me.' Then say: 'No ifs, ands or buts.' Score one point for a correct response.

7. Three-stage command
Hold out a piece of plain paper and say: 'Take the paper in your right hand, fold it in half with both hands and put it down on your lap/the table.' Score one point for each of the three correct actions.

8. Reading and obeying a command
Say: 'I would like you to read what is on this card and then do what it says. 'Show the patient a card with the words **Close your eyes** written on it. Score one point if the command is obeyed. If the subject reads the instruction but does not obey it, say: 'Now do what it says'.

9. Writing a sentence
Ask the patient to write a sentence using a pen and paper you have supplied. No prompting as to content is allowed. The sentence must contain a subject and a verb and must make sense. Score one point for a correct response.

10. Copying
Ask the patient to copy the following diagram. All ten angles should be represented and two of them must intersect; tremor and rotation are ignored. Score one point for a correct response.

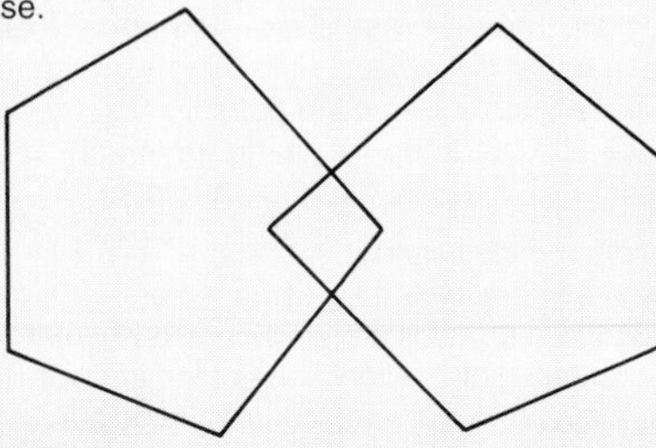

Table 2.32 (cont.)
Interpretation: the maximum score is 30. A score of 28–30 makes dementia unlikely; 25–27 is borderline, <25 is suggestive of dementia but may also occur in acute confusional states and depression.

*Reference: Folstein M. *Journal of Psychiatric Research* 1975: **12**: 189-198.

FOCAL NEUROLOGICAL SIGNS (INCLUDING STROKE)

Causes (→ Table 2.33)

Table 2.33
Causes of focal neurological deficit

Brain disorders	Stroke / TIA Epilepsy Sub-arachnoid haemorrhage Head injury Tumour or abscess Hypoglycaemia Encephalitis Subdural haematoma
Spinal cord disorders	Embolism to spinal artery (more common after surgery for aortic aneurysm) Paraspinal abscess or tumour Vertebral collapse 2° to tumour or osteomyelitis
Mixed disorders	Demyelination
Peripheral nerve disorders	Carpal tunnel syndrome Diabetes (cranial mononeuropathy) Trauma (Rarely) vasculitis

History

- The speed of onset of the deficit is important: disorders which come on instantaneously or over a few minutes are likely to be vascular in origin.
- Distribution of the weakness or sensory disturbance: involvement of the face, arm and leg on one side suggest a lesion in the internal capsule, whereas if the face alone is involved (or the face and arm), the lesion is more likely to be cortical.

Bilateral weakness, such as a paraparesis, is unlikely to be the result of a stroke.

- Ask about a past history of stroke, heart disease, hypertension, diabetes or hyperlipidaemia.
- Look for associated symptoms such as headache, mental clouding, nausea or vomiting, speech disturbance.

Examination

- If consciousness is impaired, assess conscious level formally using the GCS.
- If the patient appears to have intracranial disease (such as stroke), assess orientation (day, month, year, place) and check for the presence of dysphasia, both receptive (obeying simple commands) and expressive (naming objects).
- Examine the nervous system carefully, including sensory testing and the level of any boundary between normal and abnormal sensation.
- In the case of patients with *stroke*, check BP and examine for the presence of carotid bruits and cardiac murmurs. *Make sure you have checked for the presence of a gag reflex.*
- If the patient appears to have spinal cord disease, check perianal sensation and do a rectal examination to check sphincter tone.

Investigations

1. Check blood count, ESR, U & E and glucose. If the patient is anything other than mildly ill, these tests will need to be done urgently.
2. CXR and ECG can be ordered routinely. Syphilis serology is ordered by some teams. Check with your consultant. Skull X-ray should be requested if there is a history of trauma and X-rays of the dorsal or lumbar spine should be ordered in patients with spinal cord disorders.
3. Further investigations might include CT scan, echocardiography, bone scan, myelography or magnetic resonance imaging (MRI) scanning of the spine: consult your more senior colleagues.

Management

Stroke patients. Check the following:

- Hypertension should be treated if it is persistent, but BP should *not* be lowered rapidly unless it is causing a major problem such as papilloedema or cardiac failure. If you are tempted to lower BP rapidly, *consult a more senior colleague first.*
- Fluid should be replaced orally if possible but only if the patient has a gag reflex and can be seen to swallow water without problems. Feeding does not need to be instituted immediately but can wait until the patient can swallow or until it is clear that nasogastric feeding will be necessary.
- Good nursing care and physiotherapy are important to prevent pressure sores and contractures and to encourage mobilization. It is unwise, therefore, to lodge disabled patients with stroke on non-medical wards. Patients who are incontinent of urine may need to be catheterized in order to prevent damage to the skin.

- Patients with stroke may benefit from aspirin or anticoagulation but these should be started only after a CT scan has been done to exclude a haemorrhage as the cause of the stroke: for this reason many physicians believe that all stroke patients (except those who are likely to die quickly) should have a CT scan. If haemorrhage has been excluded, give aspirin 75–150 mg daily if the patient is in sinus rhythm; for patients in atrial fibrillation there is now good evidence that warfarin reduces future stroke risk substantially, so such patients should receive 'low-level' anticoagulation with warfarin, aiming for an INR of 1.4 – 2.8.

Paraparesis. Acute-onset paraparesis is a *neurosurgical emergency*: improvement will occur only if the spinal cord is decompressed within a few hours of the onset. Therefore in such a case, contact your SHO or registrar with a view to urgent neurosurgical referral.

Diabetic mononeuritis. This requires no specific treatment other than strict control of blood glucose. If the patient has an oculomotor weakness with diplopia, refer to an orthoptist. The patient should be warned that it may take up to 3 months for the weakness to resolve.

SECTION 3

Practical procedures

SITING AN INTRAVENOUS CANNULA

Equipment

- Cannula (17 G or 18 G)
- Tourniquet
- Cannula dressing
- Cotton wool balls
- Dressing pack
- Skin cleansing solution
- Razor (in men)
- Bag of i.v. fluid attached to giving set and run through
- 2-ml syringe containing 0.9% saline.

Procedure

1. Place the tourniquet on the upper forearm or above.
2. Inspect the arm for engorged veins: the best access point is usually the cephalic vein over the distal radius (→ Fig. 3.1). Alternatives would include more proximal branches of the cephalic vein or the median forearm vein.
3. Clean the skin well, then dry it with a cotton-wool ball or gauze. In men with hairy arms, shave the hair over a large enough area to allow the dressing to be sited on to hair-free skin.

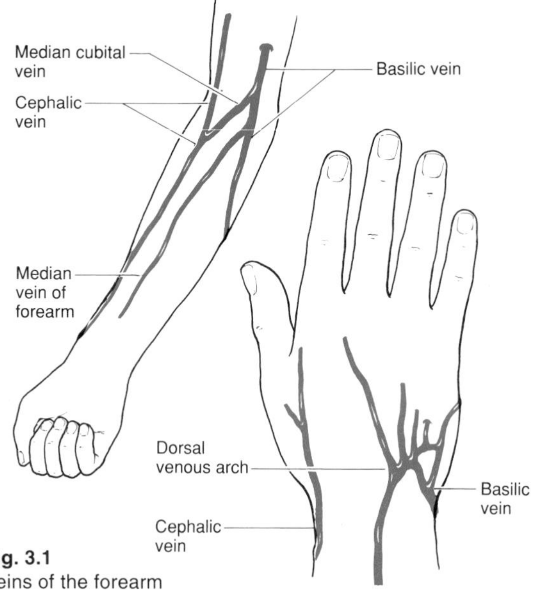

Fig. 3.1
Veins of the forearm

4. Identify an entry point, preferably where two tributaries of the vein join. Puncture the skin about 1 cm distal to the point where you plan to enter the vein.
5. Advance the needle and cannula slowly until you feel a 'give' as the needle enters the vein and until you see blood flash back into the hub of the needle.
6. Hold the hub of the needle with one hand and advance the cannula into the vein with the other.
7. If the cannula is to be used immediately for an i.v. infusion, press on the vein just proximal to the innermost end of the cannula, withdraw the needle completely and connect up the i.v. giving set. Secure the cannula in place with the dressing.
8. If the cannula is not going to be used immediately, press on the vein just proximal to the innermost end of the cannula, withdraw the needle completely and screw the screw-cap over the end of the cannula. Secure the cannula in place with the dressing. Flush the cannula with saline via the side arm.

Poor veins: place the patient's forearm in a bowl of warm water, leave for 10 minutes and try again. Alternatively, inflate a sphygmomanometer cuff on the arm to above systolic pressure and leave it in place for 2 minutes. After the cuff is released the lactic acid which has accumulated will cause reflex vasodilatation.
Fat arm: try the back of the hand (a smaller cannula may be necessary).
Fragile veins: use a smaller cannula (e.g. pink, 20 G).
Rapid infusion: if a patient needs to be given a large volume of fluid (or blood) quickly, try to insert a larger cannula, e.g. 16 G (grey).

For an i.v. infusion, insert the cannula in the patient's non-dominant arm if possible.
Do not keep on trying repeatedly if you fail to insert a cannula: two or three attempts are the most that you should allow yourself. Repeated unsuccessful attempts are distressing for the patient and may ruin those few accessible veins which the patient has. Ask someone else to do it.

Running an i.v. infusion through

It is very frustrating to try to set up an i.v. infusion if the line is full of air bubbles. Try to observe the following precautions when you run an infusion through:

1. Most i.v. giving sets are packed with the valve open, so as soon as you unpack the set, close the valve completely
2. Remove the seal on the bag of i.v. fluid and pierce it with the needle attached to the giving set. Hang the bag on a drip stand
3. Squeeze the drip chamber to bring a quantity of fluid into it (until it is about half full)
4. Hold the giving set with the far end pointing upwards and held about 6 inches below the level of the bag. Open the valve slowly and allow fluid to flow along the tube until it reaches the end.

Intradermal injections

You are unlikely to need to use this technique except for Mantoux tests and other sensitivity tests.

Method. Use a 1 ml syringe and a 25-G (brown or orange) needle. Stretch the skin between the thumb and forefinger of one hand. Holding the syringe in the other hand and with your index finger on the top of the needle hub, insert the needle at an angle of about 10° to the skin surface to a depth of about 2 mm. A raised, blanched bleb showing the tips of the hair follicles is a sign that the injection has been given correctly. (*Note:* considerable resistance is felt to a correctly given intradermal injection. If there is little or no resistance to the injection, the needle is too deep and you should withdraw it and try again.)

Subcutaneous injections

Method. Use a small syringe and a 25-G or 27-G needle. Pinch up the tissues with the thumb and forefinger of one hand and insert the needle at right angles to the skin; push the needle in up to its hilt or for a distance of 5–6 mm, whichever is the less.

Intramuscular injections

Method. Use a syringe of appropriate size for the volume of drug and a 21-G (green) needle. The injection may be given into one of three sites:

- the deltoid muscle
- middle two-thirds, lateral aspect of the thigh
- the upper, outer quadrant of the buttock (→ Fig. 3.2); it is important not to use other parts of the buttock because of the danger of injury to the sciatic nerve.

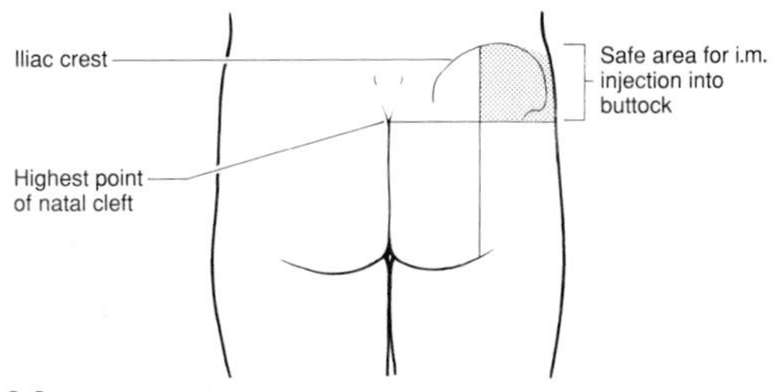

Fig. 3.2
Site for safe i.m. injection in the buttock.

Giving a local anaesthetic

Local anaesthesia is extremely effective provided that you give enough into the correct site and that you allow enough time for it to work before starting the procedure.

Method. Carry out the following:

1. Draw up 1% or 2% lignocaine into a 5 ml or 10 ml syringe (according to the procedure) using a luer filler or a 21-G (green) needle. Change to a 25-G (orange) needle and expel any air.
2. Clean the skin thoroughly. Give a small dose of lignocaine intradermally by holding the syringe with your index finger on the top of the needle hub and inserting the needle at an angle of about 10° to the skin surface to a depth of about 2 mm. A raised, blanched bleb showing the tips of the hair follicles is a sign that the injection has been given correctly. If you need to anaesthetize a large area of skin remove the needle and repeat the procedure a few millimetres away.
3. Change the needle to a 21-G (green) one. Insert the needle, at right angles to the skin, through the centre of the bleb and draw back on the piston. If no blood comes back, inject 0.1–0.2 ml of lignocaine, then advance the needle about half a centimetre, draw back again and inject another 0.1–0.2 ml. Repeat this process until you have reached the required depth. If you are going right down to bone (e.g. for an LP or chest drain insertion) try to catch the needle tip on the periosteum and inject a small volume of lignocaine under the periosteum. Remember that it is an extremely pain-sensitive structure.
4. Allow at least 3 minutes for the local anaesthetic to work before you go on. Before you proceed, test the area with a fine needle to check that anaesthesia has been successful. If not, give some more lignocaine.

Giving intravenous injections

Many drugs for intravenous administration do not come ready made up in solution but are provided in powder form, either with their own diluent or for dilution in sterile water. The bottle containing the drug is usually airtight with a rubber seal. This makes getting the diluent into the bottle (and the drug out) difficult. The following technique is recommended:

1. Draw up the required volume of diluent or water into a syringe by means of a 19-G (white) or 21-G (green) needle.
2. Put the drug bottle flat on the bench and remove the metal cap. Insert a 23-G (blue) or 25-G (orange) needle through the cap; this will act as an air vent.
3. Holding the bottle in one hand, insert the needle of the diluent syringe and inject the diluent. Do *not* inject too quickly as this may cause the solution to froth and to start coming out through the air vent.
4. Remove both needles from the bottle and shake the bottle

to dissolve the drug.

5. Draw about 3 ml of air into the syringe, invert the drug bottle and introduce the needle. Inject the air into the bottle and draw up the solution. If you start to feel resistance, pull hard, then release the piston and continue drawing up.
6. When you have drawn up all the drug, draw a couple of mililitres of air into the syringe, tip it back and forth to pick up all the little bubbles, then expel the air via the needle.
7. Check the prescription sheet to ensure that it is the right patient, the right drug and the right dose. Give the injection slowly. If especial care is needed about the speed of injection, use a watch to time yourself. If you are giving a cytotoxic drug, watch the area around the cannula entry site carefully to make sure that the drug is not 'tissuing'.
8. Inject 1 ml of sterile saline into the cannula so as to keep it patent for the next time.

TAKING BLOOD FOR CULTURE

Blood cultures need to be taken with considerable care so as to give the best possible chance of successfully isolating a pathogen and of avoiding contamination with skin commensals. Try to take the blood for culture while the patient is actually febrile.

Equipment

- Set of blood culture bottles
- 5-ml or 10-ml syringe
- 2 needles (21 G)
- Alcohol wipes.

Procedure

1. Locate a suitable vein and swab the skin over it with two or three alcohol wipes. Allow the alcohol to dry. *Do not* touch the skin again unless you are wearing sterile gloves.
2. Withdraw a suitable volume of blood (as specified on the labels of the culture bottles).
3. Change the needle and add the correct volume of blood to each bottle. *Do not overfill.*
4. Label the bottles and have them transported to the laboratory or (out of working hours) to an incubator. *Do not put them in the fridge.*

ARTERIAL BLOOD GASES (ABG)

Equipment

- 21-G (green) needle
- Pre-heparinized syringe. (If pre-packed syringes are not available you can prepare one by taking a 2-ml syringe and drawing up 0.5 ml of heparin solution, 1000 u/ml. With the heparin in the syringe and the syringe/needle pointing vertically upwards, pull the piston down to the bottom of its travel, then push it up again and expel the air. Point the needle into the sink and expel the heparin.)
- Syringe cap
- Cotton wool balls
- Drinking glass or paper cup containing ice.

Procedure

Write out the request card before you start. You do not want to waste time doing it after you have got the sample.

Radial artery. Carry out the following:

1. Lay the patient's arm comfortably on the bed or a bed-table.
2. Check that the ulnar artery is patent by compressing both radial and ulnar arteries with your fingers. Ask the patient to open and close the fist several times. Release the ulnar artery and check that the hand flushes pink.
3. Palpate the radial artery between your first and second fingers. Try to gauge both the depth and the course of the artery.
4. Keeping your index finger on the artery (but *not* compressing it!) advance the needle through the skin at an angle of 45°. Do *not* hold on to the piston of the syringe.
5. Continue advancing the syringe and needle slowly until blood flows spontaneously into the syringe. If this happens you can be sure that you have entered the artery and not a vein. If blood begins to enter the syringe but comes in very slowly, it is reasonable to apply *very gentle* traction to the piston.

> If the needle has gone into a depth of 5 mm or more but no blood has been obtained, withdraw the needle to just below the skin and advance it once again at a slightly different angle or in a slightly different direction.

6. Once you have 1–2 ml blood in the syringe withdraw the needle from the artery and apply firm pressure over the puncture site with cotton wool. Ask an assistant to maintain the pressure for at least 3 minutes.
7. Remove the needle and put the syringe cap on. Place the

syringe in the cup of ice and label the cup or the base of the syringe with the patient's name and details. Arrange immediate transport to the laboratory.

Femoral artery. Carry out the following:

1. Lay the patient flat so that the hip is in full extension.
2. Palpate the artery between your first and second fingers. Try to gauge both the depth and the course of the artery. If the pulse is difficult to feel, ask the patient to bend the knee and externally rotate the thigh.
3. Advance the needle between your fingers and through the skin at right angles to the artery. Do *not* hold on to the piston of the syringe.
4. Continue advancing the syringe and needle slowly until blood flows spontaneously into the syringe. If this happens you can be sure that you have entered the artery and not the vein. If blood begins to enter the syringe but comes in very slowly, it is reasonable to apply *very gentle* traction to the piston.

> If the needle has gone in up to the hilt but no blood has been obtained, withdraw the needle to just below the skin and advance it once again at a slightly different angle or in a slightly different direction.

5. Once you have 1–2 ml blood in the syringe withdraw the needle from the artery and apply firm pressure over the puncture site with cotton wool. Ask an assistant to maintain the pressure for at least 3 minutes.
6. Remove the needle and put the syringe cap on. Place the syringe in the cup of ice and label the cup or the base of the syringe with the patient's name and details. Arrange immediate transport to the laboratory.

Interpretation

Precise interpretation of the results of blood gases can be made by means of a Flenley diagram. However, in case you do not have one or do not know how to use it, some simple pointers are given below.

Simple hypoxia (type 1 respiratory failure). The PO_2 is less than 8 kPa (60 mmHg) but the PCO_2 is normal. This commonly occurs in lobar pneumonia or other causes of lobar collapse or consolidation (e.g. pulmonary embolism); it may also occur in asthma (though in moderate asthma the PCO_2 is usually subnormal), pulmonary fibrosis, certain kinds of chronic obstructive airways disease (especially emphysema with superadded infection), left ventricular failure.

Hypoxia with hypercapnia (type 2 respiratory failure). The PO_2 is low — less than 8 kPa (60 mmHg) — and the PCO_2 is raised (greater than 6.5 kPa; 49 mmHg). This occurs in patients with chronic bronchitis during acute exacerbations, in Adult Respiratory Distress Syndrome (ARDS), in severe pneumonia and in those with alveolar hypoventilation, e.g. Guillain-Barré syndrome.

Acidaemia (low pH) with a low PCO_2 and low plasma bicarbonate. This represents a metabolic acidosis, e.g. aspirin poisoning, diabetic ketoacidosis.

Alkalaemia (raised pH) with high PCO_2 and normal or high bicarbonate. This represents a metabolic alkalosis, e.g. prolonged vomiting.

Acidaemia with a high PCO_2, low PO_2 and high/normal or raised bicarbonate. This is an acute respiratory acidosis and is the kind of pattern you would expect to see in someone with an exacerbation of chronic bronchitis who was sick.

Acidaemia with a high PCO_2, low PO_2 and normal bicarbonate. This is an acute respiratory acidosis and is the kind of pattern you would expect to see in someone with a severe respiratory illness but who had previously been well.

Normal pH with a low PO_2, raised PCO_2 and raised bicarbonate. This represents a compensated respiratory acidosis; you would see this in someone with chronic bronchitis (i.e. a 'blue bloater') when relatively well.

Alkalaemia with a normal PO_2, low PCO_2 and normal or high/normal bicarbonate. This is a respiratory alkalosis; the commonest cause is hyperventilation.

INSERTING A CHEST DRAIN TO REMOVE FLUID OR AIR

PLEURAL EFFUSION

Symptomatic relief can often be achieved by aspirating a pleural effusion. You should observe the procedure on one or two occasions before doing it yourself and should be supervised during your first few attempts.

Equipment

- Minor dressing pack
- Gloves
- Antiseptic
- Lignocaine
- For local anaesthetic: 10-ml syringe, 21-G needle (green) and 25-G needle (blue)
- Scalpel (if inserting a drain)
- 10-ml syringe and 21-G needle (green) for a diagnostic tap
- For a therapeutic tap, a 60 ml Luer-lock syringe, 3-way tap
- 18 gauge cannula (Venflon, etc.), drainage tube and a 2-litre measuring jug to act as receiver (or one-piece, 20–24-French (Fr) G drain, with trochar, and collecting bag if the effusion is to be drained slowly)
- Specimen bottles for biochemistry (protein content), microbiology and cytology
- Sutures.

Procedure

1. Ask the patient to sit forward with the arms folded. The arms should be supported on a pillow which rests on a bed-table so that the weight of the patient's upper body is taken by the arms.
2. Percuss carefully and locate the upper limit of dullness. For a diagnostic aspiration, choose the intercostal space below this level and aim to enter it in the posterior mid-clavicular line; for a therapeutic drainage you can use the same entry site or, alternatively, a point in the 7th intercostal space mid-way between the mid-axillary and posterior axillary lines (this represents the lowest level of the pleural reflection; → Fig 3.3). Remember that you must pass through the intercostal space *above* the rib which forms its lower limit, not below the rib which is its upper limit, as the intercostal nerves and vessels run just beneath each lower rib margin.
3. Wash your hands and put on gloves.
4. Clean the skin over the entry site with antiseptic.
5. Infiltrate the skin and subcutaneous tissues with lignocaine.

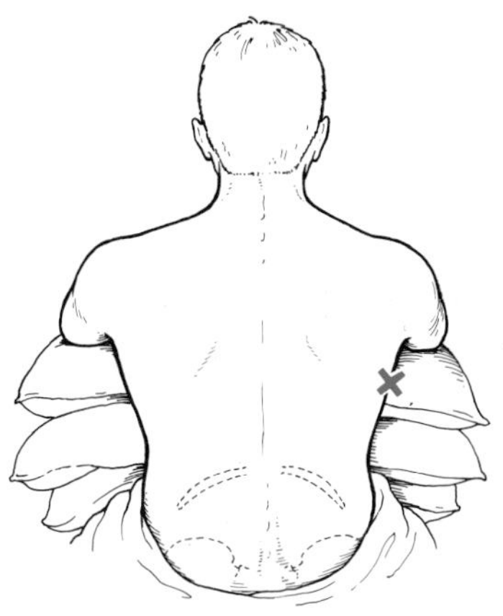

Fig. 3.3
Drainage of a pleural effusion. X marks the site for insertion of a chest drain, i.e. 7th intercostal space between the mid- and posterior axillary lines.

6. For a diagnostic tap, pass the needle through the chest wall, aspirating gently as you do so. Withdraw about 20 ml of fluid and note the colour. Remove the needle and put a dressing over the wound. Put the specimens into the respective bottles.

> Diagnostic aspirations should be done reasonably early in the day: fluid for cytology must be processed within a short time as the cells will degenerate if the specimen is kept in the fridge overnight.

7. For a therapeutic drainage, attach the cannula and 3-way tap to the syringe and introduce the needle with gentle aspiration. Once fluid is flowing freely, remove the needle, leaving the cannula in place. Attach the 3-way tap and syringe to the cannula and the drainage tube to the side arm of the 3-way tap. Ask an assistant to hold the receiver under the drainage tube. Aspirate until the fluid ceases to flow freely or until you have withdrawn 1–1.5 litres. Remember to send specimens for protein, culture and cytology. If you are leaving a drain in situ, this can be introduced using an enclosed needle or with a trochar. If you are not sure how to use this, consult someone more senior.
8. The procedure for inserting a chest drain is as follows:
   - Select a 20–24 Fr G (adult) drain and double check by dismantling and re-assembling it. Make sure that all tube connections fit correctly.

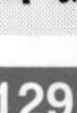

- Put the local anaesthetic into the skin (see above), then infiltrate down to the parietal pleura. Take particular care to anaesthetize the periosteum on the upper rib margin. (This whole process will require at least 10 ml of lignocaine solution.) Aspirate intermittently — withdrawal of fluid will confirm entry to the pleural cavity.
- When the local anaesthetic has worked, make an incision in the skin and subcutaneous fat: this should be less than 2 cm long so as to ensure a tight fit. Insert two loose sutures across the incision for subsequent closure after removal of the drain.
- Using blunt dissection with forceps or a scalpel, make a wide track through the muscles down to and through the parietal pleura.

> **Remember that the point of a metal trochar is not sharp enough to penetrate the muscle and pleura easily but is sharp enough to cause damage to the lung if the trochar and drain are forced into the chest.**

- Once the trochar and drain are in the pleural space, withdraw the trochar about 5 cm and advance the drain until about 5 cm are in the chest (i.e. until the point of the trochar once more approaches the chest wall). Remove the trochar and connect the drain to the drainage bag.
- Secure the drain firmly with a suture (one loop through the skin and multiple ties in at least four places on the tube itself). Loop the tube and secure it with plaster so that it cannot fall out. Prescribe adequate analgesia (oral or i.m.).

MANAGEMENT OF PNEUMOTHORAX

Pneumothorax occurs most commonly in otherwise fit young adults or in older people with chronic chest disease, chiefly emphysema. Recent guidelines (→ below) emphasize that the traditional practice of putting in a chest drain whenever a pneumothorax needed to be drained can no longer be justified: many pneumothoraces can be drained very adequately by simple aspiration.

Patients without chronic chest disease

- If the pneumothorax is *small* (a small rim of air around the lung only), drainage is not necessary.
- If the pneumothorax is *moderate* in size (lung collapsed half way towards the heart border), drainage is not necessary unless there is significant dyspnoea.
- If the pneumothorax is *large* (complete collapse of the lung), aspiration should be undertaken.
- Patients who do not require aspiration may be discharged

from hospital but should be reviewed in the chest clinic 7–10 days later. If there is any deterioration in the condition, the patient should be told to return to hospital immediately. Air travel should be avoided until the X-ray changes have resolved.

Patients with chronic chest disease

- If the pneumothorax is *small* (a small rim of air around the lung only), drainage is not necessary unless the patient is significantly more breathless than normal. However, even if aspiration is not performed the patient should be observed in hospital overnight and the chest X-ray repeated the next day. If there is no deterioration clinically or radiologically the patient may be discharged but should be given an appointment for the chest clinic 7–10 days later. If there is any deterioration in the condition, the patient should be told to return to hospital immediately. Air travel should be avoided until the X-ray changes have resolved.
- If the pneumothorax is *moderate* in size (lung collapsed half way towards the heart border) or *large* (complete collapse of the lung), aspiration should be undertaken.

Equipment for aspiration of air

- Minor dressing pack
- Gloves
- Antiseptic
- Lignocaine
- For local anaesthetic: 10 ml syringe, 21-G needle (green) and 25-G needle (blue)
- 50 ml Luer-lock syringe, 3-way tap, 16-G (or larger) cannula (Venflon, etc.), at least 3 cm long.

Procedure

1. Ask the patient to sit upright, supported on pillows.
2. Identify the entry site, usually the second intercostal space in the mid-clavicular line (fifth space in the mid-axillary line is an alternative).
3. Wash your hands and put on gloves.
4. Clean the skin over the entry site with antiseptic.
5. Infiltrate the skin and subcutaneous tissues with lignocaine; be sure to infiltrate down to the pleura.
6. Connect the 50-ml syringe and tap together. Pass the cannula/needle assembly into the pleural cavity. Remove the needle and connect the cannula to the 3-way tap.
7. Aspirate air, voiding through the side arm of the tap. Discontinue if resistance is felt, if the patient coughs excessively or if more than 2.5 litres of air have been withdrawn.

> Note that failure to aspirate sufficiently may be due to the cannula being inadvertently withdrawn from the pleural space or becoming kinked: if you suspect either of these, another attempt at aspiration should be considered.

8. Repeat CXR (departmental) in inspiration *only*. If the pneumothorax is very small or has resolved, no further drainage is required.

Once successful aspiration has been performed, a patient who was previously well can be discharged but should be asked to return to the chest clinic (→ above). Patients who have had previous chest disease, however, should be observed overnight before discharge.

INTERCOSTAL TUBE DRAINAGE

If aspiration fails an intercostal tube drain should be inserted.

Equipment

- Minor dressing pack
- Gloves
- Antiseptic
- Lignocaine
- For local anaesthetic: 10-ml. syringe, 21-G needle (green) and 25-G needle (blue)
- Scalpel
- 20–24-Fr G (adult) chest drain with trochar
- Underwater seal bottle containing sterile water
- Sutures.

Procedure

1. Ask the patient to sit upright, supported on pillows.
2. Identify the entry site, usually the second intercostal space in the mid-clavicular line (fifth space in the mid-axillary line is an alternative).
3. Wash your hands and put on gloves.
4. Clean the skin over the entry site with antiseptic.
5. Put in the local anaesthetic to the skin (→ above), then infiltrate down to the parietal pleura. Take particular care to anaesthetize the periosteum on the upper rib margin. (This whole process will require at least 10 ml of lignocaine solution.) Aspirate intermittently — withdrawal of air will confirm entry to the pleural cavity.
6. Double check the drain by dismantling and re-assembling it. Make sure that all tube connections fit correctly.
7. When the local anaesthetic has worked, make an incision in the skin and subcutaneous fat: this should be less than 2 cm long so as to ensure a tight fit. Insert two loose su-

tures across the incision for subsequent closure after removal of the drain.

8. Using blunt dissection with forceps or a scalpel, make a wide track through the muscles down to and through the parietal pleura.

The point of a metal trochar is not sharp enough to penetrate the muscle and pleura easily but is sharp enough to cause damage to the lung if the trochar and drain are forced into the chest.

9. Once the trochar and drain are in the pleural space, withdraw the trochar about 5 cm and advance the drain in an apical direction. Remove the trochar and connect the drain to the underwater seal bottle.
10. Secure the drain firmly with a suture (one loop through the skin and multiple ties in at least four places on the tube itself). Loop the tube and secure it with plaster so that it cannot fall out or kink. Prescribe adequate analgesia (oral or i.m.).

FOLLOW-UP CARE OF THE INTERCOSTAL DRAIN

Re-X-ray the patient the next day

- If the lung has re-expanded and the drain has stopped bubbling, wait 24 hours, then remove the drain (→ below). Repeat the X-ray once again: if the lung remains expanded the patient can be discharged with an appointment for the chest clinic. If, however, the lung has collapsed again, ask for help from a chest physician.
- If the lung re-expands after intubation but the drain continues to bubble, ask for help from a chest physician.
- If the lung fails to re-expand after intubation and the water in the bottle shows no bubbling or swinging, check to see if the tube has become blocked or kinked. If this has happened and the problem cannot be corrected by simple means, a new drain should be inserted through a clean incision.
- If the lung does not re-expand after intubation but there is bubbling or swinging in the bottle, ask for help from a chest physician.

If the underwater seal bottle is always kept below the level of the chest, clamping of the tube is unnecessary and potentially dangerous. As far as possible, have X-ray films taken in the department rather than on the ward; expiratory films are not necessary.

REMOVAL OF THE DRAIN

Bubbling of air should have stopped for at least 24 hours. Some patients find tube removal as traumatic as tube insertion, so consider pre-medication with atropine, 0.3–0.6 mg (to prevent a vasovagal reaction); if the patient is very anxious consider giving a small dose of intravenous midazolam (2 mg).

Equipment

- Gloves
- Stitch cutter
- Disposable sterile forceps
- Gauze pads
- Collodion
- Adhesive tape (make sure the patient is not allergic to sticking plaster).

Procedure

1. Ask a nurse to help you (you will see why lower down).
2. Scrub up and put on gloves.
3. Remove the dressing from the drain site.
4. Cut the suture which holds the drain in place with the stitch cutter and remove the suture.
5. Patients should be asked to hold their breath in maximal inspiration while the drain is removed. Tie the two sutures to seal the wound.
6. Put some collodion on a piece of gauze, apply to the wound and secure in place with tape.

Reference. Miller AC, Harvey JE (on behalf of Stand ards of Care Committee, British Thoracic Society). Guidelines for the management of spontaneous pneumothorax. *British Medical Journal* 1993; **307**: 114–116.

PASSING A URINARY CATHETER

INDICATIONS

- Monitoring urinary output, particularly peri- and post-operatively
- Acute urinary retention
- Chronic urinary retention
- Incontinence.

Catheterization of a female patient is usually performed by nursing staff, so your responsibility will usually be for male catheterization.

MALE CATHETERIZATION

Equipment

- Dressing pack
- Cleansing solution (e.g. Savlon)
- Gloves
- Drapes
- Gauze
- Lignocaine gel with sterile plastic nozzle
- Catheter (14 G)
- 20 ml syringe (luer) containing 20 ml sterile water
- 50 ml catheter syringe
- Drainage bag.

Procedure

1. Lie the patient on his back, as flat as he can manage while remaining comfortable.
2. Wash your hands and put on gloves.
3. Ask an assistant to open the dressing pack and to pour some cleaning solution into the gallipot.
4. Put sterile drapes over the patient's legs and abdomen leaving the genital area exposed.
5. Open the lignocaine gel pack and screw the nozzle onto the tube.
6. Hold the penis in your left hand using a gauze to avoid de-sterilizing your glove. Retract the prepuce fully.
7. Clean the urethral orifice and glans with antiseptic.
8. Introduce the lignocaine gel into the urethra by inserting the nozzle and then squeezing in as much of the contents of the tube as possible.
9. Hold the catheter in your right hand and ask the assistant to pull the end of the plastic wrapper off. Hold the penis vertical and insert the catheter, gently advancing it for about 3 inches; as you do this, try to withdraw the plastic

covering in stages so that the end of the cover does not touch the penis.

10. Lower the penis between the thighs and continue advancing the catheter until urine flows back down it or you have inserted about 6 inches of the catheter. *Do not* use force in advancing the catheter.
11. Once you think you are in the right place, inject about 10 ml water into the balloon via the smaller channel.

If there is any resistance or if the patient complains of pain during inflation, deflate the balloon immediately.

12. Do not forget to bring the foreskin forward again.

If urine does not flow straight away, it may be because the tip is blocked with gel. Gently aspirate the catheter using the 50 ml syringe. Alternatively, instil 20 ml sterile water into the catheter using the syringe, then gently re-aspirate.

Problems

Inability to insert. Try a smaller catheter (12 G) or a Silastic catheter (which is firmer). If you are still not successful, ask for help.

Blood draining during insertion or soon after. This is potentially a serious complication as it often means that a false passage has been created. Withdraw the catheter immediately and ask for help.

Relief of acute retention. Rapid decompression of a grossly distended bladder may lead to mucosal haemorrhage, therefore you should clamp the catheter intermittently, releasing 200–300 ml every 30 minutes. Once the kidneys have been decompressed there may be a very brisk diuresis, so observe the patient's urine output carefully and be on the look-out for dehydration.

Catheter stops draining. Ask the nursing staff to wash the catheter out with sterile water. If this does not solve the problem it is usually best to pass a new catheter.

Catheter 'bypassing'. This term is used to describe the problem of urine flowing down the urethra past a catheter in an apparently adequate position. The most common cause is catheter blockage, so ask the nursing staff to wash it out with sterile water. If this does not solve the problem, pass a new catheter. Occasionally bypassing is caused by the catheter being too small: if bypassing occurs despite the fact that urine is draining through the catheter, replace the catheter with a larger one.

FEMALE CATHETERIZATION

You will occasionally be asked to do this if the nurses have been unsuccessful. The equipment needed is the same as for male patients.

Procedure

1. Ask the patient to lie flat on her back with the knees bent up, heels together and knees widely separated.
2. Place sterile towels over the abdomen and thighs and an absorbent ('incontinence') pad on the bed between the patient's legs.
3. Separate the labia minora with your left hand and clean the vulva with antiseptic.
4. Lubricate the tip of the catheter by dipping it into sterile water, then introduce the catheter.
5. If there is a problem in isolating the external urethral meatus, e.g. in a very obese patient, ask an assistant to elevate any dependent fat from the pubic area, place the index finger of your right hand in the vagina to elevate the anterior vulva and slide the catheter along your finger (using your left hand to guide it) into the urethra.

LUMBAR PUNCTURE (LP)

Indications

1. To confirm or refute the diagnosis of:
   - sub-arachnoid haemorrhage
   - meningitis
   - Guillain-Barré syndrome
   - (rarely) neurosyphilis.
2. To administer intrathecal drugs, especially chemotherapy.

Contraindications

- Focal neurological signs
- Papilloedema
- Suspicion of a space-occupying lesion within the skull
- Severe clotting defect (including heparin or warfarin therapy)
- Major spinal deformity
- Severe contamination of the back, e.g. with dirt, faeces.

Make sure that the indication is a sound one and that there are no contraindications. If an LP is considered desirable but there is a suspicion of raised intracranial pressure, the patient must have a CT scan of the brain before the LP; this condition also applies to almost all cases of suspected sub-arachnoid haemorrhage.

Procedure

> **! You should watch several procedures before attempting LP yourself; make sure that you are well supervised when you perform your first one.**

1. LP must be carried out as a full sterile procedure.
2. Position the patient in the left lateral position with maximum flexion (→ Fig. 3.4); the back should be as close as possible to the edge of the bed. Scrub up and put gloves on.
3. Put a sterile drape over the patient's hips and another over an incontinence pad which should be placed underneath the patient.
4. Clean the skin over the lumbar spine (and a wide area around) with iodine solution (check the patient is not allergic to iodine), chlorhexidine solution or other suitable skin cleanser.
5. Feel for the highest point of the pelvic brim on the patient's right side and drop a perpendicular from here to the spine; this should bring you to the L3/L4 interspace.

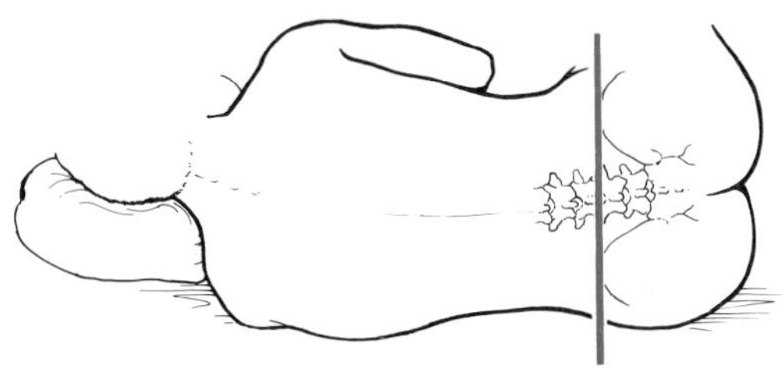

Fig. 3.4
Finding the correct site for a lumbar puncture. The line, a perpendicular from the highest part of the pelvic brim, should identify the L3/L4 interspace.

6. Palpate this interspace with the end of a finger so that you are sure where to go in with the needle.
7. Draw up local anaesthetic (lignocaine 1% or 2%) into a 10-ml syringe.
8. Fit a small (25-G) needle and inject the local anaesthetic into the skin over the planned point of entry of the LP needle. Change to a larger (21-G) needle and inject local anaesthetic into the deeper tissues.
9. Allow enough time for the local anaesthetic to work; when 3 or 4 minutes have elapsed test the skin with a needle to make sure that it is really anaesthetized.
10. Make sure that you have ready a 90-mm (18-G or 20-G) LP needle, 3-way tap, manometer, three plain sterile specimen bottles and a fluoride-oxalate (usually yellow) bottle such as is normally used for blood glucose estimation.
11. Palpate the intervertebral space again with your left hand, holding the LP needle in the right. Make sure that the stylet is fully home inside the needle and that the stud on the hub of the stylet is correctly located in the corresponding slot in the hub of the needle. Having located the correct site of entry, insert the needle with your right thumb over the end of the stylet. Advance the needle in the horizontal plane, aiming it towards the umbilicus (→ Fig. 3.5); if you hit bone or the needle seems reluctant to advance, withdraw the needle until the point is just beneath the skin and try again at a slightly different angle.

    In most adult subjects you will need to advance the needle up to at least half its length before you reach the dura; when this happens you should feel a sudden 'give' as the needle goes through the ligamentum flavum. When you feel this, withdraw the stylet to see if fluid is flowing out; if not, fully re-insert the stylet, advance the needle a few more millimetres and try again.
12. If you have reached the sub-arachnoid space CSF should flow out freely; in a healthy subject this will be perfectly clear (like distilled water). When you have a free flow, con-

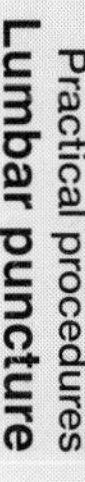

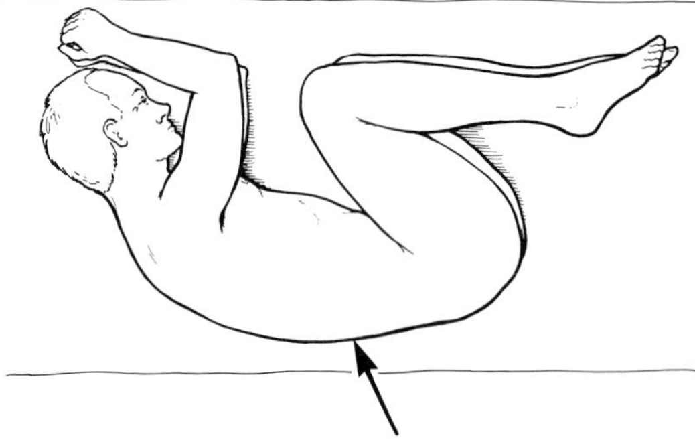

Fig. 3.5
Direction of approach for lumbar puncture. The needle is aimed towards the umbilicus.

nect the 3-way tap and manometer and measure the pressure. This should normally be between 5 and 15 cm CSF. If the pressure is very high (over 25 cm) it is customary to replace the fluid which you have sampled (see below).

13. *Queckenstedt's test*: conscious patients able to cough should be asked to do so: the pressure should rise rapidly by a further 5–10 cm, then fall rapidly back to baseline. If the patient cannot cooperate, ask an assistant to compress the root of the neck just above the medial third of the clavicle. A similar rise and fall of CSF pressure should occur with compression and release.
14. Hold a specimen bottle under the lip of the drainage tube and turn the 3-way tap to allow 1–2 ml of fluid to flow into the bottle. If the fluid is blood-stained, label this specimen as no 1 and collect two further specimens labelled 2 and 3. Finally, collect 1 ml or so of fluid into the fluoride-oxalate bottle. If the CSF pressure was very high, inject 10 ml of sterile normal saline into the needle after sampling.
15. Remove the 3-way tap and manometer and replace the stylet into the needle. Take a gauze pad in the left hand and withdraw the needle slowly with the right. Apply pressure to the puncture site with the gauze, cover with a cotton wool ball or pad then secure the dressing with tape applied over the cotton wool.

If you suspect meningitis, you must take a blood sample for glucose measurement: the CSF glucose concentration is normally about two-thirds that of the blood but will be much lower if the patient has bacterial meningitis; a value below 50% of blood glucose is abnormal. Send CSF samples for microscopy, culture, protein and glucose estimation.

16. After the procedure the patient should be nursed flat for 24 hours, otherwise there is a high incidence of headache.

INSERTING A CENTRAL VENOUS LINE

You should not attempt to insert a central venous line unless you have watched the procedure being performed at least twice. Your first few procedures must be done under supervision.

Equipment

- Sterile drapes
- Gloves
- Skin cleansing solution
- Dressing pack
- Cotton wool balls
- 5-ml syringe for local anaesthetic
- 21-G and 25-G needles
- i.v. infusion set
- 500-ml bag of 0.9% saline or 5% glucose
- Central line set with guide wire
- Ampoules of 1% or 2% lignocaine solution
- Skin suture
- Occlusive dressing ('Op-site' or 'Tegaderm').

Position of the patient

The patient should be laid flat on the back with the head supported on a single pillow. If there is any reason to suspect hypovolaemia the patient should be tilted slightly head-down so as to cause engorgement of the subclavian and internal jugular veins.

Puncture site

A central vein can be entered by a subclavian, supraclavicular or internal jugular approach. In practice, the first two are usually most suitable for patients not on an intensive care unit. It is a good idea to identify the site of entry and the approach before you scrub up.

Subclavian approach. Palpate the ends of the right clavicle and identify the centre of its lower border (→ Fig. 3.6). Your aim will be to insert the needle at this point, as close to the clavicle as possible, and to aim for the centre of the suprasternal notch.

Supraclavicular approach. Ask the patient to turn the head to the left. Palpate the junction of the sternomastoid muscle and the superior surface of the clavicle. If necessary, ask the patient to lift the head slightly off the pillow so as to make the muscle stand out. Place the middle joint of your left thumb over this junction and point the thumb backwards towards the right postero-lateral chest, bisecting the angle between the clavicle and the sternomastoid muscle (→ Fig. 3.7). The tip of your thumb will be over the entry point and you will be aiming to pass the needle in the horizontal plane, aiming for the centre of the manubrio-sternal joint.

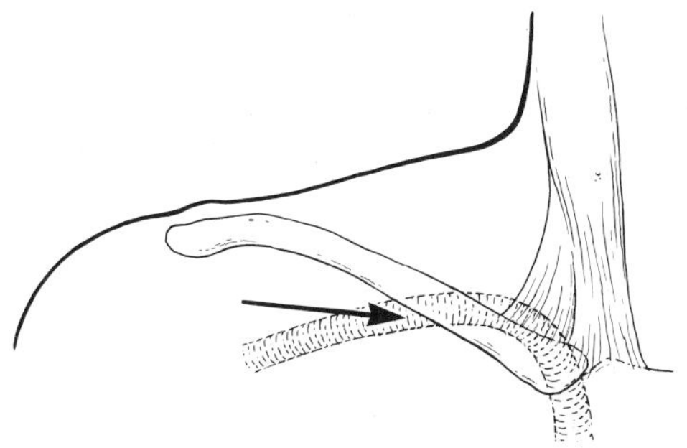

Fig. 3.6
Direction of approach for inserting a subclavian line. The needle is inserted under the mid-point of the clavicle, as close to the bone as possible, and aimed towards the middle of the suprasternal notch.

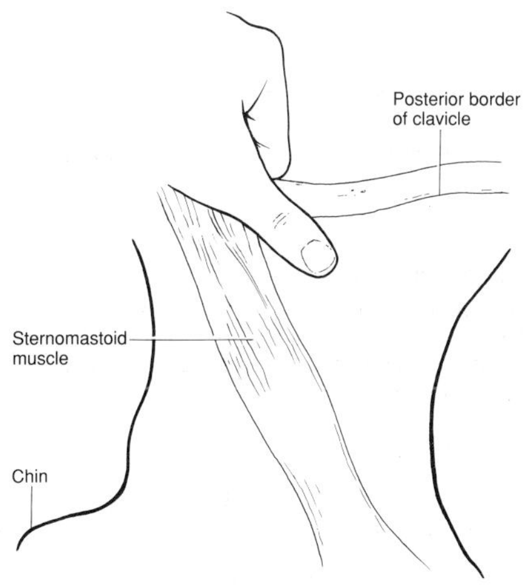

Fig. 3.7
Approach for inserting a supraclavicular line (right side). The operator stands at the patient's head and the patient looks to the left. The operator's left thumb is placed as shown, bisecting the angle between border of sternomastoid and clavicle. Tip of thumb marks the needle entry point.

Procedure

Observe strict aspesis throughout. Clean the skin and cover with sterile drapes. Identify the entry point and infiltrate with local anaesthetic. While waiting for the local anaesthetic to work, unwrap the central line and make sure that you know what all the bits do and how they fit together. Identify the 'soft' end of the guide wire. Make sure that the i.v. infusion is run through and ready to connect to the central line.

Subclavian approach. Attach the entry needle to a 10-ml syringe. Pass the needle through the skin and touch it gently against the clavicle. Direct the needle towards the suprasternal notch, keeping as close to the clavicle as you can, and apply gentle suction to the syringe as you advance. Once you enter the vein the blood should flow freely into the syringe. *If you reach the hub of the needle without having drawn blood, you have gone too far.* Withdraw the needle to just below the skin surface and advance again at a slightly different angle.

Once you have a free flow of blood into the syringe, grip the hub of the needle in one hand, remove the syringe and insert the guide wire, 'soft' end first. Advance the guide wire but *do not force it.* Remove the needle and pass the central line over the guide wire. Remove the guide wire and connect the syringe to the central line; aspirate to check that you are getting a free flow of blood back from the line. Connect the i.v. giving set to the central line and check the tightness of all connections. Secure the line in place with the skin suture and cover the wound with an occlusive dressing.

Supraclavicular approach. Attach the entry needle to a 10-ml syringe. Pass the needle through the skin and direct it, in the horizontal plane, to a point directly below the centre of the manubrio-sternal joint; apply gentle suction to the syringe as you advance. Once you enter the vein blood should flow freely into the syringe. *If you reach the hub of the needle without having drawn blood, you have gone too far.* Withdraw the needle to just below the skin surface and advance again at a slightly different angle.

Once you have a free flow of blood into the syringe, grip the hub of the needle in one hand, remove the syringe and insert the guide wire, 'soft' end first. Advance the guide wire but *do not force it.* Remove the needle and pass the central line over the guide wire. Remove the guide wire and connect the syringe to the central line; aspirate to check that you are getting a free flow of blood back from the line. Connect the i.v. giving set to the central line and check the tightness of all connections. Secure the line in place with skin suture and cover the wound with an occlusive dressing.

After insertion of the line, obtain a CXR to check for a pneumothorax and to see if the line is in the right place.

Central venous pressure (CVP)

The technique for insertion of the line is the same as that described above but, in addition to the standard equipment, you will need a CVP manometer and mounting clamp. This usually incorporates a centimetre scale and a zeroing rod containing a spirit level. The CVP manometer should be connected in line between the infusion giving set and the CVP catheter.

Before reading the CVP, ensure that the fluid being infused is 0.9% saline.

Zeroing the manometer. With the patient lying flat, align the zero mark on the manometer with a point in the mid-axillary line opposite the fourth costo-chondral junction. If the patient is lying semirecumbent, align the zero of the manometer with the manubrio-sternal joint.

Reading the CVP. With the taps turned so that the line to the patient is closed, run saline from the bag into the manometer until it is filled up to about 20 cm. Turn the taps so that the line to the bag is closed and that to the patient is open. The level of saline in the manometer should then fall freely until it reaches the level of the CVP. A normal CVP level would be: 1–8 cm measured with reference to the mid-axillary line −5 to +5 cm measured with reference to the manubrio-sternal joint.

Finally, remember to keep a very slow infusion of fluid going through the central line (of the order of 500 ml for 24 hr) in order to keep it open.

Problems with central lines

Fever. If an unexplained fever develops in someone who has a central line in situ, it is wise to consider the line as the source of the fever. Take blood cultures both peripherally and from the line. If the patient is unwell the line should be removed and the tip sent for culture; a new line can be put in if required.

Blockage of the cannula. If the line appears blocked, gently inject 10–20 ml of 0.9% saline. If this fails the line should be removed and a new one sited.

The line goes up into the neck. This happens from time to time with a subclavian approach to CVP line insertion; it is much rarer with the supraclavicular approach. Lines in this position may still be usable for drug infusion but clearly are of no value for reading the CVP; if you need a CVP reading, ask someone else to manipulate the line or to site a new one.

RECORDING AN ECG

There is a wide range of ECG machines available, most of which now have 'intelligent' controls and a range of automatic or semi-automatic functions. Routine tracings will, of course, be recorded by a cardiographer but you should make sure that you are competent at recording an ECG as you may well be expected to do so during evenings and weekends and in an emergency. Try to get a cardiographer or an experienced nurse to show you how to operate the different types of ECG machine used in your hospital. In particular you need to know:

- whether the machine should be plugged into the mains during use
- into which sockets you should plug the mains lead and the patient cable
- what type of patient electrodes to use with a particular machine
- how to switch between leads
- how to re-centre the pen in the event of baseline 'drift' (especially important for the V leads).

Procedure

1. Explain to the patient what you are going to do and that the procedure is painless.
2. Check that you have the right types of electrodes and connectors.
3. If the machine is to be used on battery only, check that it is charged up.
4. Attach the limb electrodes to the patient, using plenty of electrode gel if using plate electrodes. Try to attach to hairless areas of the limbs. The connecting wires are usually labelled and/or colour-coded, the most widely used convention for the colours being: *red* – right arm, *yellow* – left arm, *green* – left leg, *black* – right leg.
5. Palpate the intercostal spaces and attach the chest electrodes (→ Fig. 3.8). (In men with hairy chests you may have to shave the hair off the left side of the chest in order to get good electrical contact).
6. Check that the machine is set to 10 mm per mV and to a paper speed of 25 mm/sec.
7. Ensure that the patient is comfortable and is lying still. Set the paper in motion and mark a calibration mark.
8. Record the ECG, making sure to keep the tracing in the centre of the paper. If the patient has an arrhythmia, record a long rhythm strip (at least 10 complexes) in lead II or V1, depending on which is giving you the better signal.
9. Label each lead as soon as you have finished it and label the whole tracing with the patient's name and the date and time of recording: nothing is more frustrating than finding an ECG tracing lying around the notes trolley and not being able to identify the patient to whom it relates or

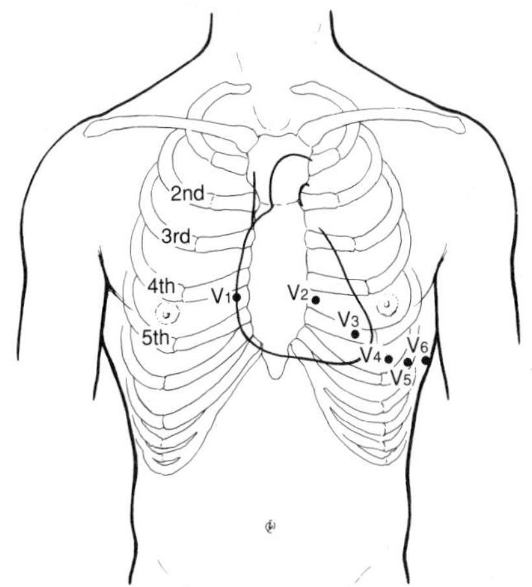

Fig. 3.8
Positions of the chest electrodes of the ECG. Note that V5 and V6 are in the same horizontal line as V4, not the same intercostal space.

the date and time of the recording.

10. Remove the electrodes from the patient and clean off the gel. Remember to clean well under the left breast in the case of well-endowed women. Clean or wash the electrode plates, coil the cables up neatly and put them away.
11. Do not forget to tell the patient what the ECG has shown and to provide appropriate re-assurance.

Common ECG patterns

Figures 3.9–3.20 illustrate the common rhythm disorders. Patterns for MI are shown in Figures 5.1 – 5.4 (→ p 219).

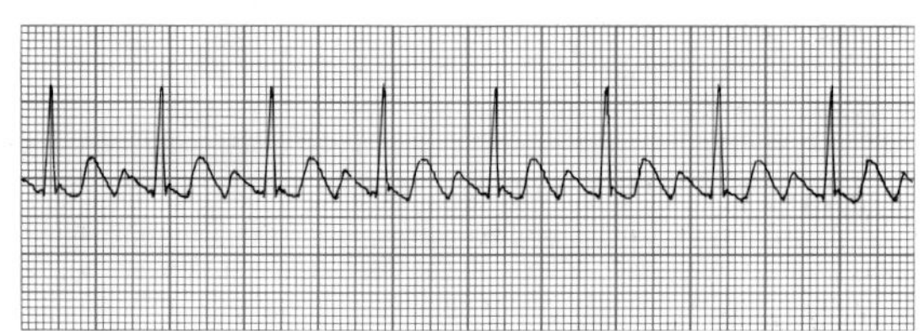

Fig. 3.9
Atrial flutter.

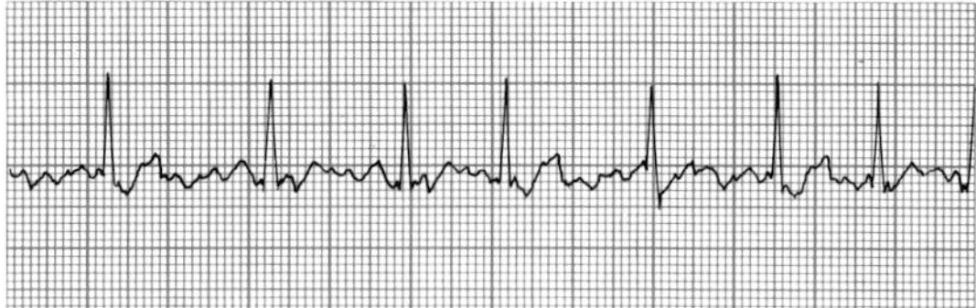

Fig. 3.10
Atrial fibrillation.

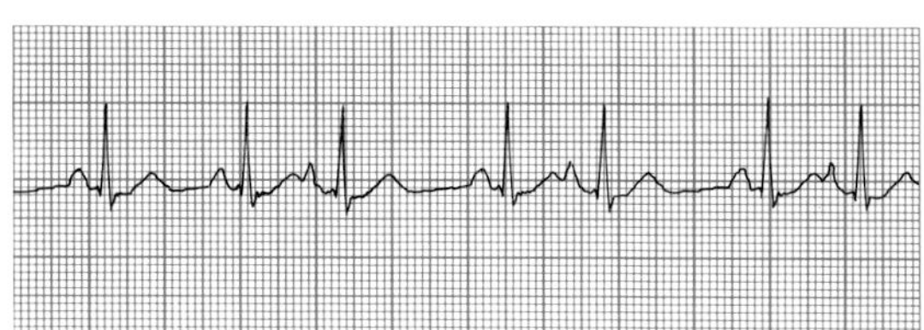

Fig. 3.11
Atrial ectopics.

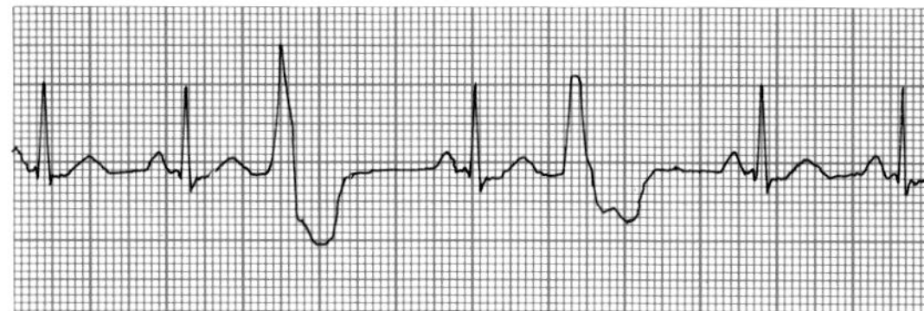

Fig. 3.12
Ventricular ectopics.

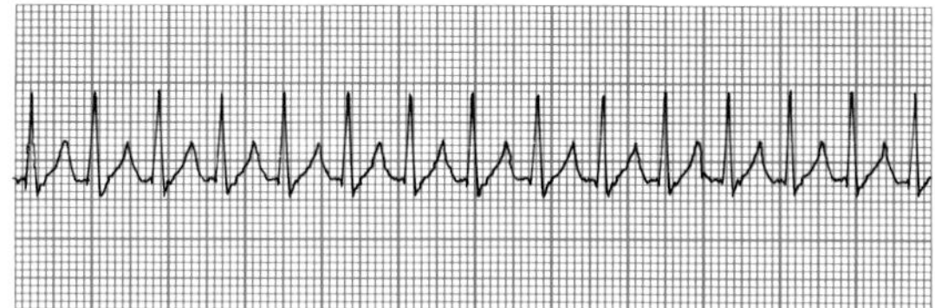

Fig. 3.13
Supraventricular tachycardia.

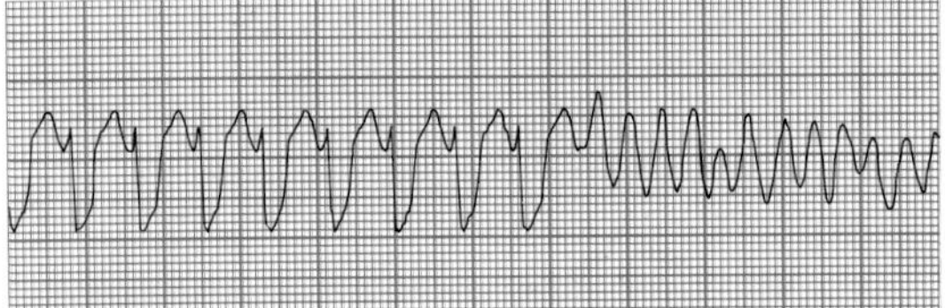

Fig. 3.14
Ventricular tachycardia and fibrillation.

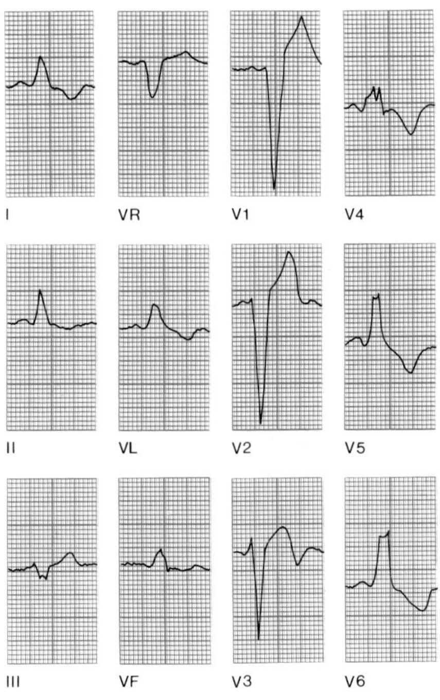

Fig. 3.15
Left bundle branch block.

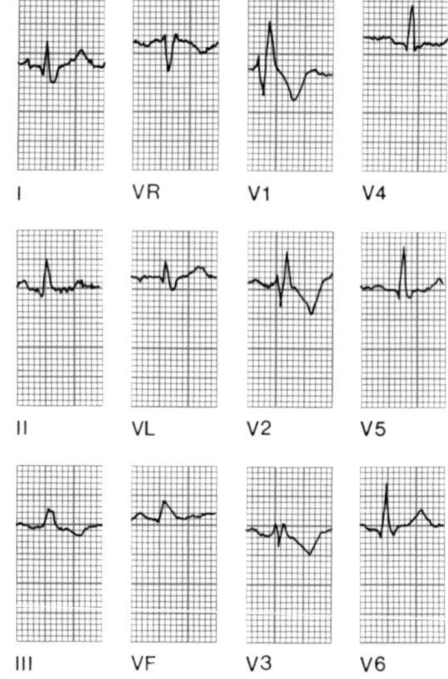

Fig. 3.16
Right bundle branch block.

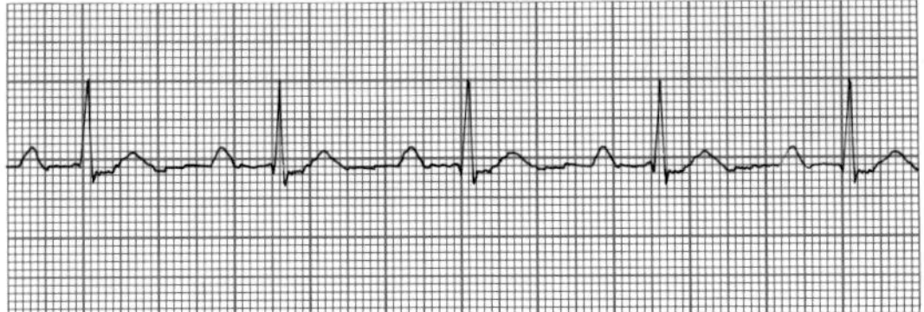

Fig. 3.17
First degree heart block.

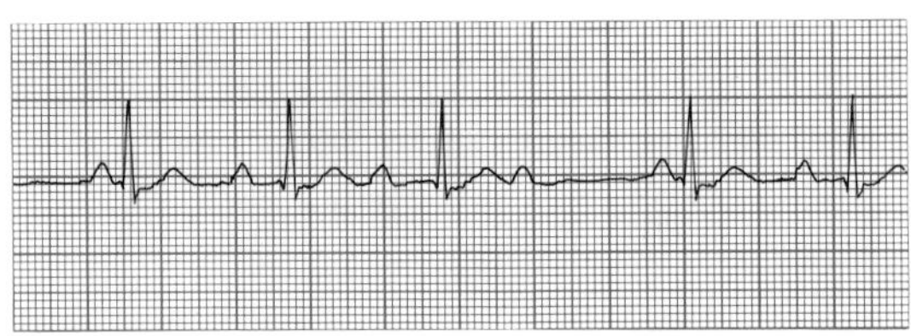

Fig. 3.18
Second degree heart block (Mobitz type I or Wenckebach)

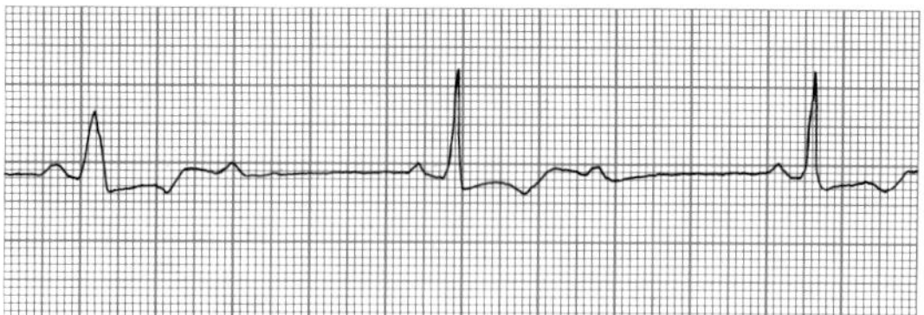

Fig. 3.19
Second degree heart block (Mobitz type II).

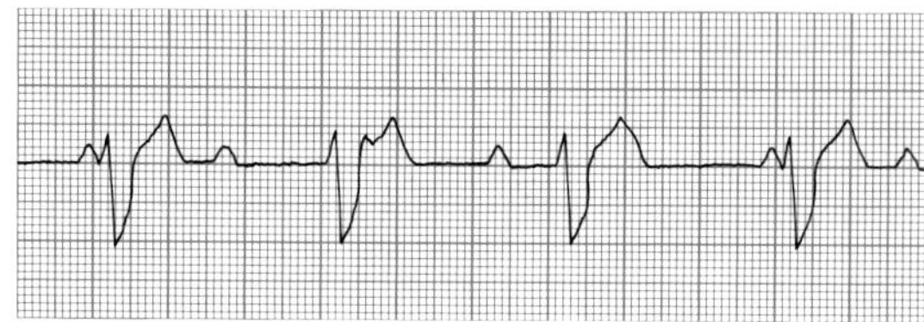

Fig. 3.20
Complete (third degree) heart block.

INTRAVENOUS FLUIDS

The regulation of electrolyte and water balance is a function of the kidneys (with contributions from some other organs). Intravenous fluid therapy can be thought of as providing the kidneys and other vital organs with an adequate blood flow.

The normal distribution of body water and electrolytes

The body water is contained in two compartments, the intracellular fluid (ICF) and the extracellular fluid (ECF); the ECF is further subdivided into fluid within the blood vessels and circulation (intravascular) and fluid outside the vessels (tissue or interstitial fluid). The capillary endothelial membrane, which separates the intravascular fluid from the interstitial fluid, is permeable to water, ions and certain small molecules. The amount of fluid in the various compartments is shown in Fig. 3.21.

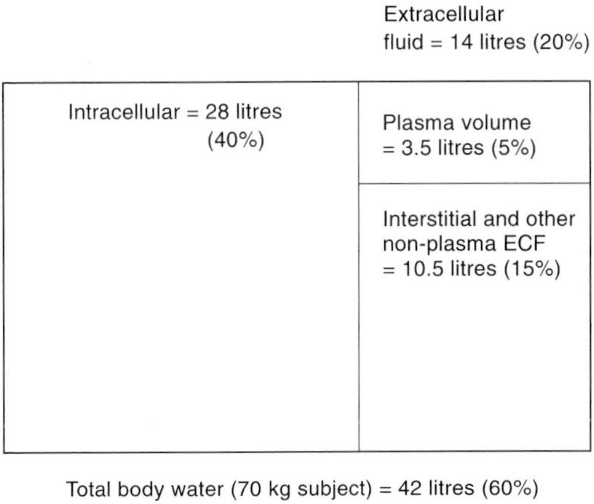

Fig. 3.21
Body fluid compartments. Volumes are for a 70 kg man; % figures are percentages of total body weight.

The term 'electrolytes' includes sodium, potassium, chloride and bicarbonate. Water can diffuse freely through all of the fluid compartments but electrolytes cannot move freely in and out of cells. The electrolytes make up the major solutes in the body fluids and account for most of the osmotic pressure.

The total osmotic activity of plasma is normally 285 – 295 mOsmol/kg water and most of this activity is provided by sodium and chloride, with a small amount from bicarbonate, potassium, urea, glucose, other minerals and proteins.

The osmotic pressure of the interstitial fluid differs from that of the plasma only by the contribution of plasma protein; this is about 1.5 mOsmol/kg and exerts a 'pull' which is roughly equivalent to a hydrostatic pressure of 25 mmHg.

Movements of fluid

Fluid moves because of a hydrostatic or osmotic gradient across a membrane. The plasma contains crystalloids (electrolytes, etc.), which pass freely across the capillary membrane, and proteins, to which the membrane is not freely permeable. Thus the plasma proteins, albumin and globulins, are in high concentration within the vascular compartment (60–80 g/l) whereas protein concentrations in the interstitial fluid are much lower (7–20 g/l). The osmotic pressure produced by proteins is called the colloid osmotic pressure (COP); about 75% of the COP of plasma is due to albumin (MW 69 000), the rest to globulins.

Thus fluid flow across capillary membranes depends on:

- the filtration properties of the capillary wall
- the hydrostatic pressure inside the capillary and the COP of the plasma
- the hydrostatic pressure and the COP in the interstitial fluid.

The electrolytes (sodium and potassium)

Sodium is maintained largely as an extracellular ion while potassium is mainly intracellular. The average daily intake of sodium in temperate climates is around 100–300 mmol; an amount almost equal to this is lost each day in the urine. The normal intake of potassium is 50–80 mmol; most of the excreted potassium is lost in the urine but a small amount passes out in sweat and faeces. There is also an active secretion of potassium by the colonic mucosa. Because potassium is mainly an intracellular ion, plasma levels may not reflect overall potassium balance. Potassium is lost from the cells into the plasma, and then into the urine, whenever water is mobilized, as during water deprivation or uncontrolled diabetes, and when cell protein is broken down. It is actively secreted by the distal renal tubules. Conversely, renal impairment often leads to accumulation of potassium, sometimes with severe and life-threatening hyperkalaemia.

Causes of potassium depletion (→ Table 3.1)

Table 3.1
Causes of potassium depletion

Losses in the urine	Diuretic therapy, osmotic diuresis of diabetes, primary renal disease (occasionally)
Drugs other than diuretics	Steroids, salbutamol, insulin (during acute treatment of diabetic emergencies)
GI losses	Chronic diarrhoea (e.g. ulcerative colitis), excessive use of purgatives, malabsorption syndromes, villous adenoma of the rectum

Hypokalaemia and potassium depletion can cause cardiac arrhythmias and muscular weakness. Hypokalaemia is especially dangerous in patients receiving digoxin.

FLUIDS AVAILABLE FOR REPLACEMENT

Fluid can be given in the form of crystalloids, colloids or blood. Crystalloids can pass freely through the capillary membrane, i.e. between the circulation and the interstitial fluid. Colloids contain large molecular weight substances which cannot escape from the plasma (unless it is flowing through damaged capillaries), so they are chiefly retained in the circulation.

Water balance (→ Table 3.2)

Table 3.2
The daily water balance

Output (ml)		Intake (ml)	
Lungs	500	Oral fluid	1700
Skin	900	Food	1000
Faeces	100	Metabolic water	300
Urine	1500		
Total	3000	Total	3000

The alimentary tract secretes a substantial volume of fluid (some 8 litres) into its lumen each day (→ Table 3.3).

Table 3.3
Volume of fluid secreted by alimentary tract

Saliva	1.5 l
Gastric juice	2.5 l
Small intestinal fluid	3.0 l
Bile	0.5 l
Pancreatic juice	0.7 l

The changes in the volume of fluid are important in patients with GI disease or paralytic ileus.

The crystalloids

The contents of each litre of solution are summarized in Table 3.4.

Table 3.4
Contents of litre of crystalloid solution

	Normal saline	5% Glucose	Glucose/saline	Hartmann's
Sodium	150 mmol		30 mmol	135 mmol
Chloride	150 mmol		30 mmol	
Glucose		50 g		

Osmolality: 300 mmol/l for all the above

Potassium chloride is usually added at 2 g/l (27 mmol/l of potassium)

Colloids

These solutions are used to support the circulation in hypovolaemic shock before blood is available or when it is not needed. They can also be used to 'bulk up' red cell concentrates, which may have as little as 40 ml of the original plasma per unit. Albumin solution is the natural colloid which one might think of using but it is expensive and should only be used in carefully selected cases (→ see below). In most cases when a colloid is needed, one uses gelatins (Gelofusin, Haemaccel), synthetic colloids such as dextrans (e.g. Dextran 70, Macrodex, Lomodex) or modified starch such as hetastarch (Hespan). The properties of these colloid solutions are summarized in Table 3.5.

Table 3.5
Properties of colloid solutions

Dextran 70	
Half-life in circulation:	12 h
Maximum dose:	20 ml/kg
Colloid osmotic pressure:	268 mmHg
Cost per 500 ml:	£4
Special features:	Has an anticoagulant effect but interferes with blood cross-matching, so a sample must be taken for this before beginning treatment with Dextran 70
Haemaccel	
Half-life in circulation:	5 h
Maximum dose:	30 ml/kg
Colloid osmotic pressure:	350 – 390 mmHg
Cost per 500 ml:	£3
Special features:	Contains much more calcium than Gelofusin. This may cause clotting in warming coils when Haemaccel is mixed with citrated blood or FFP
Gelofusin	
Half-life in circulation:	4 h
Maximum dose:	30 ml/kg
Colloid osmotic pressure:	465 mmHg
Cost per 500 ml:	£3
Special features:	Useful for rapid fluid volume replacement (→ below)
Hespan	
Half-life in circulation:	17 days
Maximum dose:	ad libitum
Colloid osmotic pressure:	?
Cost per 500 ml:	£16
Special features:	Very slowly eliminated from the body

FLUID ADMINISTRATION

The amount of fluid administered will depend on:

- projected fluid needs over the next 12 – 24 hours
- whether the patient is fluid overloaded, dehydrated or in balance.

As mentioned above (→ p155), a subject who is adequately hydrated will lose 2500 – 3000 ml per day (i.e. 100 – 125 ml per h) as the result of urinary losses (1500 ml), respiratory losses (500 ml) and evaporation from the skin (500 – 1000 ml). This is therefore the basic fluid requirement of a subject who cannot take any food or fluid orally. There may be additional losses due to fever, diarrhoea, GI fistulae, intestinal obstruction, etc.

Assessment of state of hydration. This is based on clinical and biochemical evidence. Examination of skin turgor (over the chest wall, not the arm) can be misleading in the elderly or where there has been weight loss. Early evidence of hypovolaemia is provided by peripheral vasoconstriction, i.e. pale, cool extremities and empty peripheral veins. Another useful sign is postural hypotension: if the systolic BP drops by 25 mm or more when the patient sits up from a lying position, or if it falls below 90 mm then hypovolaemia is probably present. In young adults, however, there may be no helpful physical signs because of sympathetic compensatory mechanisms.

Evidence of volume depletion. This usually takes the form of a rise in blood urea and haematocrit, though care must be taken to allow for pre-existing renal disease or anaemia. As regards urinary measurements, the most helpful information is related to urine volumes per unit time and to urine specific gravity. If possible, body weight should be measured daily since, in the short term, changes in body weight are a good guide to net gain or loss of fluid. If clinical or biochemical evidence of volume depletion is present then there is probably a deficit of at least 5% of total weight (i.e. 3 – 4 l). These observations do not always quantify the deficit but they do give essential information against which to control replacement.

Deficit corrections. How fast the deficit is corrected depends on its severity: hypovolaemia resulting in oliguria must be rapidly corrected, with hourly assessments of progress.

While preparations are being made for urgent surgery 2 – 4 hours are usually available; the first litre of normal saline can be given in 30 minutes and a second in 60 minutes; subsequent infusion rates will depend on the clinical response and on the need for potassium. (Serum potassium levels below 3.5 mmol/l are not favoured by anaesthetists!) In the absence of oliguria it is sensible to replace the fluid deficit over 12 – 24 hours (or even 48 hours in patients over 70). The main hazards of over-rapid rehydration are left ventricular failure, hyponatraemia and cerebral oedema.

Dangers of colloid solutions. Many artificial colloid solutions contain substantial quantities of sodium which may cause problems in patients with cardiac or renal failure or with liver disease (→ below).

Patients may display allergic reactions to colloid solutions; in the event of a serious reaction the infusion should be stopped and adrenaline, 5 – 10 ml of 1:10 000 by slow intravenous injection or 0.5 – 1 ml of 1:1000 by i.m. or s.c. injection should be given immediately. Adrenaline injections should be repeated every 15 minutes until improvement occurs. The patient should also be given hydrocortisone, 100 – 200 mg intravenously and, because of circulatory collapse, will need large volumes of crystalloid (1–2 l).

Prescribing i.v. fluids

All intravenous fluids must be prescribed and signed for. The prescription will state the volume, the nature of the fluid and the rate of infusion; this rate is adjusted by counting the drop rate. A standard giving set in the UK delivers 15 drops to a ml and an infusion rate of 20 drops per minute will deliver 960 ml in 8 hours.

Fluid balance should be assessed each morning and the fluid requirements for the next 24 hours prescribed. This should be re-assessed in the afternoon and adjusted on the basis of the measured fluid balance and laboratory results.

TYPE OF FLUID

The normal requirement of 2500 ml per day can be provided as 1000 ml of 'normal' (0.9%) saline and 1500 ml of 5% glucose or as 2500 ml of glucose saline (dextrose/saline); these fluids will also supply the required 75 –100 mmol of sodium.

Supplementary potassium

Potassium chloride is added to the standard solutions at a concentration of 2 g per litre (27 mmol/l); thus 2.5 litres will supply 68 mmol of potassium. Stronger infusions of potassium are sometimes indicated: in hypokalaemia infusion rates of up to 20 mmol per hour may be needed. At higher infusion rates (over 10 mmol per h) you should consider ECG monitoring. Infusion at more than 20 mmol per hour is hazardous (risk of cardiac arrest) and should only be undertaken, if at all, with the agreement of a senior colleague. If a concentrated solution of potassium is to be infused, precautions *must* be taken to avoid over-rapid infusion, i.e. the infusion must be controlled by the use of an automatic, programmable infusor (e.g. an IMED device) or a paediatric burette. When adding potassium chloride to a bag, remember that it is denser than the rest of the fluid and the bag must be shaken before use. An additive label must also be filled in and affixed to the bag before it is connected to the patient.

FLUID REPLACEMENT IN SPECIFIC SITUATIONS

Blood loss: upper GI haemorrhage, trauma or during surgery

The gelatins (e.g. Haemaccel, Gelofusin) are effective short-term plasma substitutes and large volumes can be infused without impairing haemostasis. They have a short half-life so blood or plasma can be given soon after with less risk of fluid overload. Up to 1500 ml of blood loss can be replaced by gelatin; between 1500 and 4000 ml blood loss replacement should be with equal volumes of gelatin and blood. For losses over 4000 ml the ratio should be two parts blood to one part gelatin. The haematocrit should not be allowed to fall below 25%. Some patients with sepsis, severe trauma, liver disease or malignancy will have abnormalities of blood clotting such as DIC. If you are in any doubt about the integrity of the patient's clotting mechanisms, check platelet count, PT, KCCT/APTT and fibrinogen titre. If the clotting times are prolonged the patient may need FFP, vitamin K or platelet transfusion. Ask advice before giving these items.

Practical points about blood transfusion

- Use a large-bore cannula wherever possible.
- When setting up an i.v. infusion, begin by infusing a small amount of normal saline to make sure that the line is flowing freely; do not use dextrose as it will cause the line to clog.
- Give whole blood for the treatment of acute haemorrhage; packed cells for the treatment of anaemia.
- Give each unit over 4 hours, or more rapidly if the patient is actively bleeding or hypotensive. Consider giving 20 mg of frusemide orally or i.v. with the second and subsequent units (especially in the elderly). Start the transfusion early in the day: patients need frequent observations during a transfusion and if this is given overnight the patient will not get much sleep.
- Check the haemoglobin 24–48 hours after transfusion.

Hypovolaemia and dehydration

Water and electrolyte deficiency. This may result from many causes, e.g.:

- diarrhoea and vomiting
- overdiuresis
- nausea and vomiting due to vestibular disease
- dysphagia due to oesophageal disease or cerebrovascular accident (CVA)

• septic shock
• burns.

As a general rule crystalloid (saline or glucose solution) should be used initially. A subject who is adequately hydrated will lose 2500 – 3000 ml per day (i.e. 100 – 125 ml per h) as the result of urinary losses (1500 l), respiratory losses (500 ml) and evaporation from the skin (500 – 1000 ml). This is therefore the basic fluid requirement of a subject who cannot take any food or fluid orally. The dehydrated patient, will need 1000 – 2000 ml of fluid per day over and above this basic requirement, i.e. a total of 3500 – 5000 ml per day (150 – 200 ml/h). If, in order to restore normal hydration, more than 5 litres are required the addition of colloid may be beneficial. If the patient has cardiac or renal disease or is elderly it may be better to give fluid at the rate of 1500 – 2000 ml per day (60 – 80 ml/h) or, if dehydrated, 2500 – 3000 ml per day (100 – 125 ml/h).

Acute pancreatitis. The mainstay of treatment is correction of hypovolaemia by replacement of fluid and electrolytes by infusion of crystalloids as above (→ p 156). Fluid sequestration in the first 48 hours may amount to 6 litres, necessitating large positive fluid balances. In some cases blood or plasma may be needed.

Diabetic ketoacidosis and other diabetic emergencies. (→ p 236–237).

Fluid deficit in adult respiratory distress syndrome (ARDS) and anaphylaxis

In these conditions, where plasma colloid osmotic pressure is low or the capillaries are leaky, a mixture of crystalloid and colloid should be used in roughly equal amounts (for rates of fluid administration → p 158).

Use of albumin

Albumin is indicated in the treatment of diuretic-resistant oedema in hypoproteinaemic patients. Hypoproteinaemia of any cause leads to contraction of the intravascular volume, which leads to compensatory retention of water and sodium. If a patient does not respond to diuretics, albumin together with intravenous diuretics and an aldosterone antagonist will usually produce a diuresis. Albumin is not effective as parenteral nutrition. The available albumin solutions are summarized in Table 3.6.

Table 3.6
Albumin solutions

Plasma protein fraction (stable plasma protein solution)	
Albumin concentration	50 g/l
Colloid osmotic pressure	26 – 30 mOsm/kg
Sodium concentration	140 –160 mmol/l
Potassium concentration	Less than 2 mmol/l
Human albumin solution 5%	
Albumin concentration	40 – 50 g/l
Colloid osmotic pressure	26 – 30 mOsm/kg
Sodium concentration	140 – 160 mmol/l
Potassium concentration	Less than 2 mmol/l
Human albumin solution 20%	
Albumin concentration	200 g/l
Colloid osmotic pressure	100 – 120 mOsm/kg
Sodium concentration	140 – 160 mmol/l
Potassium concentration	Less than 10 mmol/l

BLOOD TRANSFUSION

INDICATIONS FOR WHOLE BLOOD TRANSFUSION

Whole blood should be given to patients who are actively bleeding or who have recently lost blood.

Procedure

1. Take blood for FBC, serum iron or ferritin, B_{12} and folate and cross-match *before* giving any blood. *Take great care* over labelling the sample on the cross-match form. Mistakes in this area are potentially fatal.
2. If the patient is severely shocked, ask for group O, Rh negative blood, which you can give to the patient before the cross-match has been completed. If the patient needs blood quickly but is not actually shocked (e.g. someone who has had a large haematemesis but who is maintaining a systolic BP of >100 mmHg), ask for grouped, uncrossmatched blood (grouping takes far less time than a full cross-match).
3. Give the blood at a rate of one unit every half an hour unless the patient's clinical state indicates a need to give blood more rapidly. During transfusion the patient's temperature, pulse and BP should be checked every half hour.

> **! Blood cannot be given simultaneously with glucose solutions, nor should it be given into a line which has just been used for glucose infusion; the glucose causes red cell agglutination. If you need to give blood into such a line, flush it with 10 ml normal saline first.**

INDICATIONS FOR TRANSFUSION OF PACKED RED CELLS

Packed cells are given for the correction of anaemia. Only in very rare circumstances is it justifiable to transfuse someone whose anaemia has not been investigated (→ p 36–38); transfusion may, however, be undertaken while the results of tests are awaited. Transfusion is usually carried out if the haemoglobin concentration is less than 7 g/dl or the patient is very symptomatic. As a general rule, each unit of packed cells will raise the haemoglobin concentration by about 1 g per dl.

Procedure

1. Take blood for FBC, serum iron (or ferritin), B_{12} and folate *before* giving any blood. *Take great care* over the labelling of

the sample and the cross-match form, as mistakes in this area are potentially fatal.

2. Give blood at the rate of one unit every 3–4 hours. Do not give routine transfusions after 10 p.m. The frequent nursing observations which the patients will require mean that they will get very little sleep!

If the patient is elderly or has a history of heart disease, transfusion should be performed under diuretic cover: give 20 mg of frusemide orally or i.v. with every alternate unit.

TRANSFUSION REACTIONS

A low-grade fever (less than 39°C) is relatively common in a patient receiving a transfusion and, if the patient is otherwise well, is not a cause for concern. However, if during a transfusion the patient develops one or more of the following:

- high fever (>39° C) ± rigors
- urticarial rash
- hypotension
- wheezing
- severe back pain

then it is likely that you are dealing with a transfusion reaction. In that case you should:

1. stop the transfusion and return the rest of the unit to the laboratory
2. give 100 mg of hydrocortisone and 10 mg of chlorpheniramine i.v.
3. if the patient is unwell or is getting worse *inform your SHO or registrar urgently*
4. ask the laboratory to re-check the cross-match between the patient's and the donor's blood
5. monitor urine output carefully (if necessary, catheterize the patient). There is a risk of acute renal failure.

Other complications of blood transfusion

- Transmission of infection, e.g. hepatitis.
- Hyperkalaemia (stored red cells tend to leak potassium into the fluid phase).
- Hypocalcaemia due to the action of the anti-coagulant; this may be a practical problem if the volume transfused has been particularly large (more than 8 units).
- Thrombocytopaenia : platelets do not survive for long in stored blood. This rarely causes a practical problem except in patients whose platelet count is already low (e.g. those with leukaemia or aplastic anaemia).

- Clotting factor depletion: this rarely causes a clinical problem except in those whose clotting was already severely damaged (e.g. severe liver disease). Clotting factor replacement should *not* be undertaken routinely just because the patient has had a large-volume blood transfusion but may be required if laboratory measures show a severe coagulation defect.

PLATELET TRANSFUSIONS

These may be required in patients who have severe thrombocytopaenia, e.g. those with leukaemia or aplastic anaemia. The level of the platelet count is, on the whole, *not* a good guide to the need for a platelet transfusion, but transfusion is indicated if any of the following apply:

- There is spontaneous bruising/bleeding into the skin or optic fundi, from venepuncture sites, etc.
- The platelet count is less than 20×10^9/litre.
- The patient requires surgery and the platelet count is less than 50×10^9 per litre.

If you do decide to give platelets, give four or (preferably) six units as a rapid infusion.

Fresh frozen plasma (FFP)

This is given to correct deficiencies in clotting factors.

Indications for FFP transfusion. The major indications are:

- warfarin overdosage with moderate or severe bleeding (INR usually greater than 5)
- liver disease with coagulation disorder (both clinical and on laboratory tests)
- DIC.

If you do give FFP, give either 2 or 4 units as a rapid infusion.

> ↘ FFP is expensive and carries all the hazards of blood transfusion. It should not be used simply as a source of plasma proteins or as a volume expander.

SECTION 4

Drug prescribing

INTRODUCTION

The range of drugs available to doctors is very large and continues to grow; no attempt will be made, therefore, to describe them all here. Before prescribing any drug with which you are unfamiliar, you are strongly encouraged to consult the current edition of the BNF or the manufacturer's data sheet. It is especially important that you do this before prescribing anything for a patient who is already on several drugs, for a pregnant or nursing mother or for someone with liver or renal disease.

The following sections cover the drugs which are most commonly prescribed by house officers.

DRUGS FOR ACUTE PAIN

ANALGESICS

An analgesic is given to relieve pain and also to keep pain at bay. Therefore if a patient requires painkillers, on an as-required basis, more often than twice in a day, consider the following questions:

- Are you confident that you understand the cause of the pain?
- Should the patient have regular analgesia (every 4 or 6 hours, say) rather than p.r.n. (as required) treatment?

Aspirin and paracetamol

These are the drugs that should almost always be used first; most patients know which drug suits them best.

Dose. Adults: aspirin — 600 mg every 4–6 hours
paracetamol—1 g every 4–6 hours.

Co-proxamol

This compound is frowned upon by pharmacologists as controlled trials have failed to show superiority over paracetamol. Many clinicians, however, believe that it is more effective than paracetamol alone, presumably because of a mild euphoriant effect of the dextropropoxyphene.

Dose. Adults: 2 tablets 4–6 hourly (minimum dose interval 4 h).

Codeine and dihydrocodeine

These are more powerful than the above but have a higher incidence of side-effects, especially constipation and, in the case of dihydrocodeine, nausea and vomiting.

Dose. Adults: 30–60 mg 4–6 hourly. In some instances it is useful to combine a small dose of codeine with paracetamol, using a combined preparation such as Tylex (paracetamol 500 mg plus codeine phosphate 30 mg) or co-codamol (paracetamol 500 mg plus codeine phosphate 8 mg); the dose is 1–2 tablets or capsules every 4–6 hours (maximum 8 per day).

Non-steroidal anti-inflammatory drugs (NSAIDs)

Ibuprofen is the mildest; dicoflenac, naproxen, ketoprofen, etc. are of medium strength; indomethacin is the most powerful. These are useful drugs for such things as muscular, joint or skeletal pain and also for pericarditis. Increased potency goes hand-in-hand with increased side-effects, notably dyspepsia and frank peptic ulceration (+/− perforation or bleeding). The value of topical NSAID gels is controversial. NSAIDs should be used with great caution in the elderly as they can cause fluid retention (thereby precipitating heart failure) and because of an increased incidence of side-effects.

Dose. Adults: ibuprofen — 400 mg 3 times daily
diclofenac — 75–150 mg daily in 2–3 divided doses; 100 mg by suppository
naproxen — 500–1000 mg daily, usually in divided doses
indomethacin — 50–200 mg daily in divided doses.

Buprenorphine

This drug, given sublingually, is an effective and relatively safe form of pain relief. It causes less respiratory depression than morphine but its effects are only partly reversed by naloxone. It commonly gives rise to nausea or vomiting.

Dose. Adults: 200 μg 8 hourly, increased to a maximum of 400 μg 6 hourly.

Pethidine

Given by injection, pethidine is an effective but short-acting opiate analgesic.

Dose. Adults: 25–100 mg; may be repeated after 4 hours.

Morphine sulphate

This drug can be very useful in acute pain and, in short-term use, does not cause serious problems with dependence. It can be given in liquid form and by suppository. Nausea, drowsiness, constipation and psychological disturbance are common side-effects. Modified-release formulations such as MST Continus are *not* suitable for acute pain relief.

Dose. Adults: 10–20 mg every 4 hours if given by mouth or by s.c. or i.m. injection; for i.v. use, 5–10 mg doses should be used.

Diamorphine

This is the drug of choice for severe pain, e.g. in MI or aortic dissection. Nausea is very common and diamorphine is routinely given along with an anti-emetic such as prochlorperazine (12.5 mg) or metoclopramide (10 mg). Diamorphine is usually given by s.c., i.m. or i.v. injection or infusion.

Dose. Adults: 5 mg every 4 hours (occasionally 10 mg in larger subjects). In MI, give a further 2.5 mg if the initial dose has not been effective after 15–20 minutes.

THE 'ANALGESIC LADDER'

Doctors are fairly successful at treating acute pain but are often criticized by patients with chronic pain for prescribing drugs which are too weak and for prescribing them too infrequently, often because of misplaced fears of dependency or addiction. Therefore, if you are treating a patient with chronic pain, do not continue with a particular analgesic for more than 48 hours unless it is successfully controlling the pain; if not, move up to the next step on the 'analgesic ladder' (→ Table 4.1) and consider combinations of drugs with different modes of action (e.g. a mild opiate plus an NSAID).

Table 4.1
The 'analgesic ladder'

Step 1	Aspirin, paracetamol
Step 2	Mild opiates (codeine, dihydrocodeine)
Step 3	NSAIDs
Step 4	Strong opiates (morphine, diamorphine, etc.)

The basic principles of treating chronic pain can be summarized briefly as follows:

- Give an analgesic which fully suppresses the pain, wherever possible.
- Give analgesics orally wherever possible.
- In terminal illness, be prepared to give very large doses of opiates if that is what is needed to control pain.
- Give analgesics frequently enough to prevent pain re-emerging: it is easier to keep the patient comfortable if pain is suppressed rather than if one has to treat repeated episodes of 'breakthrough' pain.
- If the patient is needing frequent doses of oral morphine, especially in malignant disease, consider using a modified-release morphine tablet such as MST Continus. For example, if someone has needed 120 mg of oral morphine in the last 24 hours, this could be given as one 60 mg tablet every 12 hours.

Modified-release morphine *must not* be given more frequently than every 12 hours.

- If the patient cannot take oral treatments, an i.v. or s.c. continuous infusion of analgesic is kinder and more effective than intermittent injections. One can also combine the analgesic with an anti-emetic in the same syringe: thus one can combine diamorphine, 10–20 mg with hyoscine, 800 µg or methotrimeprazine, 50 mg, in a small volume (10–20 ml) of 0.9% saline and infuse the mixture s.c. over 24 hours; the dose of either component can be increased if needed.

- Remember other forms of treatment for pain such as radiotherapy (for bone metastases), steroids (for liver metastases), transcutaneous electrical nerve stimulation, local heat.
- If you or a nurse can find time to talk to patients about pain and their illness generally, this will ease a lot of the distress associated with the pain.
- Many hospitals have staff with expertise in managing severe or persistent pain such as anaesthetists who run pain clinics or, in the case of malignant disease, Macmillan nurses. Do not feel reluctant to refer your patient to one of these specialist services.

Prescribing of controlled drugs

The law on the prescribing of controlled drugs for use outside hospital is very strict. So, for example, if you are prescribing a controlled drug on a TTO prescription, you *must* observe the following rules:

- **The entire prescription, including the patient's name and address, must be in the doctor's own handwriting.**
- **The form of the drug (tablet or elixir) must be stated, together with the strength.**
- **The total amount of the drug to be dispensed must be stated in *words and figures*.**
- **The prescription must be signed and *dated* in the doctor's own handwriting.**

Controlled drugs regulations apply to all opiate analgesics except codeine and dihydrocodeine, and also to many barbiturates, notably amylobarbitone, butobarbitone, quinalbarbitone and, in a slightly less severe form, phenobarbitone. If in doubt, check with the BNF.

ANTI-ANGINAL DRUGS

Nitrates

Glyceryl trinitrate. This is a safe and effective drug for the acute relief of anginal pain. It can be given as a sublingual tablet or as a buccal spray: the tablets, once the bottle is opened, have a limited life (8 weeks); the spray has a longer life but is more expensive. Nitrates frequently cause headache and can, in large doses, cause faintness.

Dose. Acute attack: 1–2 sublingual tablets or doses of spray, repeated as required.

Glyceryl trinitrate can also be given in sustained release forms, including a buccal tablet (held between the gum and upper lip) such as Suscard; a patch form for transdermal administration is also available. These long-acting forms are useful for preventing angina but must *not* be given continuously: a break in therapy of 6–8 hours in 24 is necessary to sustain clinical benefit.

Dose. Suscard Buccal: 1–5 mg 3 times daily
nitrate patch: 5–10 mg once daily.

In severe angina, glyceryl trinitrate can be given intravenously (→ below).

Long-acting oral nitrates. These are effective in preventing angina. There are a wide variety of preparations available, with differing lengths of action, and it is best to become familiar with one or two of them. Both isosorbide dinitrate and mononitrate are marketed; choice is largely a matter of personal preference, though current fashion seems to be in favour of the mononitrate. These drugs should *not* be given continuously throughout the 24 hours: a break in therapy of 6–8 hours is necessary to sustain clinical benefit. For this reason, if one is giving the drug b.d., the second dose should be given in the early afternoon.

Dose. Isosorbide mononitrate: 10 mg b.d. for 3 days, then 20 mg b.d., increased as necessary. Maximum 120 mg per day
Isosorbide mononitrate (modified release): 30–60 mg once daily, increased to 120 mg once daily if needed.

In unstable or severe angina, nitrates can be given *intravenously* in the form of glyceryl trinitrate (e.g. Nitronal) or isosorbide dinitrate (e.g. Cedocard IV or Isoket).

All intravenous nitrates should be given using glass or polyethylene apparatus: loss of potency will occur if polyvinylchoride (PVC) is used.

Headache and hypotension are important side-effects of i.v. nitrates, so begin with a small dose (1–2 mg per hour, depending on the size of the patient) and increase the dose every half hour until either the pain is fully controlled or the systolic BP falls below 100 mmHg. Maximum dose 10 mg per hour.

Beta-blockers

These are highly effective anti-anginal drugs but there are many side-effects and contraindications. There are a large number of beta-blockers on the market so try to become familiar with just two or three of them.

Absolute contraindications. These include: known hypersensitivity to these drugs; a history of asthma; heart block; bradycardia; hypotension; heart failure.

Relative contraindications. These include: peripheral vascular disease; insulin-dependent diabetes; chronic liver or renal disease (depending on the drug); late pregnancy.

Side-effects. These include: breathlessness (due either to bronchospasm or to heart failure); bradycardia; hypotension; lethargy; nightmares, GI disturbances; impotence.

Dose.

atenolol:	25–100 mg daily
metoprolol:	50–100 mg 2–3 times daily
oxprenolol:	40–160 mg 3 times daily
labetalol:	50–100 mg twice daily initially, increased to 400 mg twice daily or to a maximum of 2.4 gm daily in 3–4 doses
sotalol:	80 mg twice daily initially, maximum 600 mg per day
bisoprolol:	5–10 mg once daily; occasionally 20 mg daily.

Sotalol has the advantage compared with other beta-blockers, that it also possesses some class III anti-arrhythmic activity, i.e. it is a 'poor man's amiodarone'.

Calcium channel blockers

These drugs are effective anti-anginal agents with a better adverse-effect profile than beta blockers, though they tend to be more expensive. The number of drugs and formulations continues to increase, so try to become familiar with two or three of them.

Absolute contraindications. These incluse: known hypersensitivity; advanced aortic stenosis; pregnancy. Verpamil and diltiazem are also contraindicated in the presence of bradycardia, sick sinus syndrome, any degree of heart block, cardiogenic shock or a history of heart failure.

Relative contraindications. These include: hepatic or renal impairment; abrupt worsening of angina after starting therapy. Verpamil is usually contraindicated in the acute phase after MI because of the risk of precipitating heart failure.

Side-effects. These include: constipation; nausea and vomiting; flushing; headache; fatigue; ankle oedema; hypotension; bradycardia; heart failure; depression.

Dose. For acute anginal attacks: Nifedipine 5–10 mg (the patient should bite into the capsule and then swallow it).
For angina prophylaxis:

nifedipine retard	— 10–40 mg twice daily
verapamil	— 80–120 mg 3 times daily
verapamil sustained release	— 120–240 mg once or twice daily
diltiazem	— 60–120 mg 3 times daily
diltiazem sustained release	— 90–180 mg once or twice daily or 300 mg once daily.

Aspirin

This is a useful addition to anti-anginal therapy if a patient's pain is not adequately controlled despite several other drugs.

Absolute contraindications. These include: known hypersensitivity; peptic ulceration; bleeding disorders.

Relative contraindications. These include asthma; uncontrolled hypertension; recent stroke (if patient has not had a CT scan).

Side-effects. These are uncommon at low dosage but can include bronchospasm, dyspepsia, GI haemorrhage.

Dose. 75–300 mg once daily.

Heparin

This drug can be added to the treatment of patients with unstable angina who are not responding well to other treatment. It should be given intravenously in conventional anticoagulating doses (→ p208).

Summary (→ Table 4.2)

Table 4.2 Summary of treatment of unstable angina.
Bed rest
Beta-blockade (unless contraindicated)
Aspirin
i.v. nitrate
Calcium antagonist
Heparin
Consider early exercise testing and/or coronary angiography

DRUGS FOR HEART FAILURE

Left ventricular failure (LVF) (manifested by pulmonary oedema) may be present without audible crackles in the chest and vice versa. If you are in any doubt, therefore, about the need for anti-failure treatment it is wise to arrange a CXR.

DIURETICS

For mild heart failure a thiazide diuretic such as bendrofluazide or hydrochlorothiazide may be adequate. More severe degrees of heart failure will require loop diuretics such as frusemide or bumetanide; in the most severe cases the loop diuretics will be best given intravenously. In chronic heart failure of moderate or severe degree, metolazone (a very powerful drug, especially if combined with frusemide) may be useful, sometimes on an intermittent basis (alternate days or even once a week).

Potassium supplements or potassium-sparing drugs need not be given routinely with thiazides: a slight fall in serum potassium (to between 3.0 and 3.5 mmol/l) is usually clinically insignificant. Hypokalaemia is, however, dangerous in people with severe coronary atherosclerosis or a history of ventricular arrhythmias and in patients taking digoxin. Many patients taking loop diuretics will require potassium replacement but in any case such patients should be having regular measurements of serum potassium. For medium to long-term use, combined tablets containing a diuretic together with a potassium-sparing drug are often useful; examples would include Moduretic and Dyazide (thiazide plus potassium-retaining drug), Frumil, Frusene, Burinex A and Aldactide (loop diuretic plus potassium sparing drug).

Thiazides

Contraindications. These include: diabetes mellitus; pregnancy; hyperuricaemia.

Side-effects of thiazides. These include: hypokalaemia; impotence, hyponatraemia; hypomagnaesaemia; hyper-uricaemia; hyperglycaemia.

Doses.

bendrofluazide	— 5–10 mg daily
hydrochlorothiazide	— 25–100 mg daily
Moduretic	— between one tablet of 'moduret 25' daily and 2 tablets of moduretic twice daily
Dyazide	— 1–3 tablets daily.

Moduretic users have a high incidence of hyponatraemia, sometimes severe.

Loop diuretics

Absolute contraindications. These include: known hypersensitivity; severe liver failure.

Relative contraindications. These include: pregnancy; diabetes mellitus; gout; severe liver disease.

Side-effects. These include: hypokalaemia; hyponatraemia; hypotension; nausea; muscle cramps; glucose intolerance; hyperuricaemia; (in large doses) tinnitus or deafness.

Dose.

Oral:	frusemide	— 40 mg once daily to 80 mg twice daily; higher doses in renal failure
	bumetanide	— 1–2 mg daily; up to 5 mg daily in resistant cases
	metolazone	— 5 mg once a week to once daily, usually as an adjunct to a loop diuretic; higher doses needed occasionally.

If you are giving someone more than 80 mg per day of frusemide (or 2 mg daily of bumetanide) for heart failure, you should consider changing the patient to an ACE inhibitor, either alone or in combination with a diuretic.

Dose.

Combined oral preparations:	Frumil —	1–2 tablets daily or twice daily
	Burinex A —	1–2 tablets daily
Intravenous:	frusemide —	20–50 mg as initial treatment in an emergency; dose should be given over 5 min.

	— 40–160 mg daily in subacute or chronic severe heart failure
bumetanide	— 1–2 mg as initial treatment in an emergency
	— 1–4 mg daily in subacute or chronic heart failure.

ANGIOTENSIN CONVERTING ENZYME (ACE) INHIBITORS

There is increasing evidence that ACE inhibitors are effective treatments for heart failure, not simply in relieving symptoms but also in improving cardiac performance and survival. These drugs are therefore being introduced at an earlier stage in the management of heart failure than they used to be. There are now 8 ACE inhibitors available in the UK and the number may increase further, so try to become familiar with just two or three drugs.

Absolute contraindications. These include: known hypersensitivity; known or suspected renal artery stenosis; aortic stenosis or outflow tract obstruction; pregnancy; severe hypotension.

Relative contraindications. These include: renal failure; recent high-dose diuretic therapy.

Side-effects. These include: persistent dry cough; loss of taste; sore throat; hypotension; hyperkalaemia; proteinuria; rashes; worsening renal impairment; neutropenia or thrombocytopenia; liver damage.

If a patient is being treated with a diuretic together with an ACE inhibitor, it is not usually necessary to give supplements of potassium or a potassium-retaining drug.

Dose. Initiation of ACE inhibitor therapy is best done in hospital if the patient is on large doses of diuretics or has a low BP (less than 130 mmHg systolic). If the patient is on a large dose of diuretic (more than 80 mg frusemide or 2 mg bumetanide per day) this should, if possible, be stopped for 24 hours before introducing an ACE inhibitor. To initiate therapy, give a single dose of 6.25 mg captopril while the patient is lying down. Ask the nurses to measure the BP every $\frac{1}{4}$ hour for 2 hours, then $\frac{1}{2}$ hourly for 2 hours, then hourly. If the systolic pressure remains above 90 mmHg and the patient has no symptoms of faintness, ACE inhibition can be safely continued: begin regular treatment with captopril, 6.25 mg 3 times daily, increased as needed to a maximum of 25 mg, 2–3 times daily. Once the patient is established on ACE inhibition, it may be simpler to transfer to a longer-acting agent such as enalapril, 5–20 mg daily or lisinopril, 5–20 mg daily.

Renal function must be closely monitored during the early stages of ACE inhibitor therapy.

VASODILATORS

These may be useful in the treatment of heart failure where ACE inhibitors are contraindicated, are not tolerated or are insufficient.

Nitrates

These have a useful effect in heart failure. There are a wide variety of preparations available, with differing lengths of action, and it is best to become familiar with one or two of them. Both isosorbide dinitrate and mononitrate are marketed; choice is largely a matter of personal preference, though current fashion seems to be in favour of the mononitrate. These drugs should *not* be given continuously throughout the 24 hours: a break in therapy of 6–8 hours is necessary to sustain clinical benefit. For this reason, if one is giving the drug b.d., the second dose should be given in the early afternoon.

Dose. Oral: isosorbide mononitrate — 10 mg b.d. for 3 days, then 20 mg b.d., increased as necessary. Maximum 120 mg per day
isosorbide mononitrate (modified release) — 30–60 mg once daily, increased to 120 mg once daily if needed.

In severe heart failure nitrates can be given *intravenously*, either in the form of glyceryl triniterate (e.g. Nitronal) or isosorbide dinitrate (e.g. Cedocard i.v. or Isoket).

All intravenous nitrates should be given using glass or polyethylene apparatus: loss of potency will occur if PVC is used.

Side-effects of i.v. nitrates. The most important are headache and hypotension.

Dose. Begin with a small dose (1–2 mg per hour, depending on the size of the patient) and increase the dose every half hour until either the failure is fully controlled or the systolic BP falls below 90 mmHg. Maximum dose 10 mg per hour.

Hydrallazine

This drug is only effective if given together with a diuretic.

Absolute contraindications. These include: systemic lupus erythematosus; severe tachycardia; cor pulmonale; aortic stenosis or outflow tract obstruction; dissecting aortic aneurysm; recent MI.

Relative contraindications. These include: renal impairment; coronary artery disease; cerebrovascular disease; pregnancy or breast feeding.

Side-effects. These include: tachycardia; fluid retention; nausea; headache; SLE-like syndrome; hypotension.

Dose. Adults: 25 mg twice daily, increased if necessary to 50 mg daily.

Prazosin

This drug has a better side-effect profile than hydralazine but hypotension is an important problem.

Absolute contraindications. These are unknown apart from previous hypersensitivity to the drug and hypotension.

Relative contraindications. These include : renal impairment; tendency to postural hypotension.

Side-effects. These include: postural hypotension; drowsiness; lack of energy; headache; nausea; palpitations; urinary frequency.

Dose. Adults: 0.5 mg at bed-time, followed by 0.5 mg 2–4 times daily, increased to 4 mg daily in divided doses.

DIGOXIN

The beneficial affects of digoxin in heart failure are weak and short lasting. It should only be used on rare occasions and then only after consultation with your seniors.

INOTROPIC AGENTS

Intravenous inotropes are useful in certain patients with acute, severe cadiovascular disease associated with hypotension, e.g. cardiogenic shock. You should *not* initiate treatment with an inotrope without consulting a more senior colleague.

Dobutamine

This drug is effective but its use may be limited by tachycardia: a ventricular rate above 140/min reduces cardiac filling and tends to cancel out the benefit of the positive inotropic action. The drug is given in *diluted form* and the manufacturers supply a 'ready reckoner' chart to help you work out the dose.

Make sure that both you and the nurse supervising the infusion understand the chart.

Dose. Adults: 2.5–10 μg/kg/minute; occasionally doses up to 20 μg may be used.

Dobutamine should not be discontinued abruptly; the dose should be reduced gradually over 24–48 hours.

Enoximone

This drug works by a different mechanism from that associated with dobutamine. There are no absolute contraindications to enoximone.

Relative contraindications. These include: outflow tract obstruction; renal impairment.

Side-effects. These include: ectopic beats or other arrhythmias; hypotension; headaches; insomnia; nausea and vomiting, diarrhoea.

Enoximone must always be infused into a central vein.

Dose. Adults: 90 μg/kg/min initially, followed by 5–20 μg/kg/min
Total dose in 24 hours should not exceed 24 mg/kg.

ANTIHYPERTENSIVE DRUGS (pp 46–49)

DRUGS FOR TACHYCARDIA

SUPRAVENTRICULAR TACHYCARDIAS (SVT)

There is no ideal drug for treating SVT, particularly paroxysmal SVT. The choice of drug will depend on safety, side-effects and the preferences of your superiors.

Digoxin

This is the drug of choice for the control of tachycardia in atrial fibrillation. It has many potential toxic effects and a narrow 'therapeutic window' (i.e. the effective dose is close to the toxic dose).

Absolute contraindications. These include: severe hypokalaemia; Wolf-Parkinson-White syndrome.

Relative contraindications. These include: hypokalaemia; renal failure, hypothyroidism.

Side-effects. These include: anorexia; nausea and vomiting; diarrhoea; confusion; ventricular arrhythmias; heart block. Side-effects are more likely in the elderly and in patients who are hypokalaemic or who have pre-existing myocardial or conducting-system disease.

Dose. Adults: Oral — 250–750 μg initially, followed by 250 μg 6 hours later; maintenance dose 62.5–500 μg per day, in 1 or 2 doses

i.v. — 750–1000 μg diluted in 50 ml of 5% glucose and infused over 2 hours, followed by maintenance doses as above.

Digoxin levels in blood. Blood for digoxin assay must be taken 6 or more hours after the last dose. Levels *cannot* be used to fine-tune the dose of digoxin which a patient needs, nor does a level within the 'therapeutic range' exclude the possibility of digoxin toxicity. A very low level suggests that the patient may not be taking digoxin consistently, while a level at or above the top of the range indicates a high risk of toxicity.

> Patients who are seriously ill due to digoxin toxicity should be treated with digoxin monoclonal antibodies (Digibind). The dosage is complex and depends on the blood level of digoxin, so consult the manufacturer's data sheet.

Verapamil

This drug is very effective, given intravenously, for the acute termination of SVT. It is much less satisfactory for chronic, oral use as its effectiveness tends to wane with the passage of time. It is sometimes useful, as an adjunct to digoxin, for the control of rapid atrial fibrillation.

Absolute contraindications. These include: hypotension; sick sinus syndrome; history of heart failure or left ventricular (LV) dysfunction; recent beta-blocker therapy; Wolf-Parkinson-White syndrome.

Relative contraindications. These include: hepatic impairment; pregnancy; acute MI. You should not give verapamil to someone with a broad-complex arrhythmia unless you are quite sure that it is not ventricular tachycardia.

Side-effects. These are rare with acute i.v. use but can include: nausea and vomiting; flushing; headache; heart failure.

Dose. i.v. with ECG monitoring: 5–10 mg given slowly; a further 5 mg may be given 10 minutes later if required.

Disopyramide

This drug is effective, both intravenously and orally. It impairs myocardial contractility but probably less so than verapamil.

Absolute contraindications. These include: glaucoma; prostatic enlargement; liver or renal impairment; pregnancy; old age.

Side-effects. These include: myocardial depression; hypotension; atrioventricular block; dry mouth; blurred vision; urinary retenion.

Dose. Oral: 100 mg 3 times daily, increased to 200 mg 4 times daily if needed. May also be given in modified-release form (Dirthymin SA or Rythmodan Retard) every 12 hours.

i.v. with ECG monitoring: 100 mg slowly over 5 minutes, followed immediatel by 200 mg orally; may also be given by i.v. infu sion at a rate of 0.4 m g / kg/h to a maximum of 300 mg in the first hour.

Some physicians use a combination of verapamil and disopyramide to bring about a 'medical cardioversion' for patients in atrial fibrillation. You should *not* use this cocktail unless you have first discussed it with your SHO or registrar, nor should you use it if there is any risk of precipitating heart failure. The usual practice is to give a dose of 5 mg verapamil slowly, followed by 100 mg disopyramide over 5 minutes. **The verapamil must always be given first.**

Esmolol (beta-blocker)

Esmolol, a very short-acting beta-blocker, is useful for the acute treatment of SVT.

Absolute contraindications. These include: asthma; obstructive airways disease; heart failure; cardiogenic shock; sick sinus syndrome.

Relative contraindications. These include: late pregnancy; liver disease; renal disease; insulin-dependent diabetes; peripheral vascular disease.

Dose. Adults: 50–200 μg/kg/minute by i.v. infusion. Consult data sheet.

Sotalol (beta-blocker)

Sotalol is useful for the treatment of SVT because it possesses class III anti-arrhythmic properties as well as its beta-blocking action. Contraindications are the same as for esmolol; there is also a risk of ventricular arrhythmias so it is **particularly important to avoid hypokalaemia**.

Side-effects. These include: breathlessness (due either to bronchospasm or to heart failure); bradychardia; hypotension; lethargy; nightmares; GI disturbances; impotence.

Dose. Adults: 20–240 mg daily, in 1 or 2 doses.

Amiodarone

This is an extremely effective anti-arrhythmic drug. It does not cause as much myocardial depression as other anti-arrhythmic drugs. It can be used for both supraventricular and ventricular arrhythmias. It has many potential toxic effects.

Absolute contraindications. These include: sinus node or sino-atrial disease; pregnancy and breast feeding; (for i.v. use) severe respiratory failure; severe hypotension; severe cardiac failure; thyroid dysfunction; iodine sensitivity.

Relative contraindications. These include: renal impairment; cardiac failure; old age.

Side-effects. These are numerous and sometimes serious. They include: peripheral neuropathy; myopathy; bradycardia; potentiation of the effects of digoxin (which should be stopped or reduced when amiodarone is being given); phototoxicity; hypo- or hyperthyroidism; pulmonary alveolitis; hepatitis; headache.

Dose. Oral: 200 mg 3 times daily for a week, then 200 mg twice daily for a week, then 100–200 mg daily
i.v.: 1200 mg by infusion over 24 hours. The initial dose is usually 5 mg/kg, given over 30 min followed by the remainder of the 1200 mg over the succeeding 23½ hours.

Amiodarone infusion must always be given via a central venous catheter.

Adenosine

This is a short-acting drug which can be used in several types of SVT, including those associated with Wolff-Parkinson-White syndrome. It can also be used in a diagnostic test for broad-complex tachycardias (those which respond are supraventricular in origin).

Absolute contraindications. These include sick sinus syndrome; second- or third-degree atrioventricular (AV) block.

Relative contraindications. These include: atrial flutter or fibrillation in patients with an accessory pathway; concurrent or recent treatment with disopyramide.

Side-effects. These include: facial flushing; dyspnoea; choking sensation; nausea; light headedness; severe bradycardia (requiring pacing).

Dose. Adults: Given into a large peripheral vein by rapid injection — 3 mg, followed if necessary by 6 mg 1–2 minutes later and by 12 mg after a further 1–2 minutes.

Quinidine

This is a rather old-fashioned drug but it is effective, particularly in paroxysmal SVT. There are, however, a number of potential side-effects.

Absolute contraindication. Heart block.

Side-effects. These include: nausea; diarrhoea, rashes; myocardial depression; heart failure; thrombocytopenia; ventricular arrhythmias; haemolytic anaemia.

Dose. Adults: 200 mg test dose to detect hypersensitivity, then 500 mg every 12 hours, given as a modified-release preparation (Kiditard or Kinidin Durules).

Flecainide

This is a powerful drug with 'broad-spectrum' anti-arrhythmic activity. Its use has recently been linked, however, with ventricular arrhythmias which appear to be *caused* by the drug. For this reason you should never use it except with detailed advice from a senior colleague.

VENTRICULAR TACHYCARDIAS (VT)

Ventricular ectopic beats rarely require treatment: although they have been claimed to predict more serious arrhythmias there is no evidence that treatment of ectopics improves survival, no matter how 'serious' they look on the ECG monitor. Drug treatment is therefore restricted to ventricular tachycardia (VT); the diagnosis and the management of VT can be very difficult so you are advised to consult your SHO or registrar.

Lignocaine

This is the first-line drug for the suppression of VT.

Absolute contraindications. Theses include: sino-atrial or atrio-ventricular block; severe heart failure.

Relative contraindications. These include: congestive cardiac failure; liver failure.

Side-effects. These are: confusion; convulsions.

Dose. Adults: 100 mg intravenously over 2–3 min followed by 4 mg per min by i.v. infusion.

Amiodarone

This is an extremely effective anti-arrhythmic drug. It does not cause as much myocardial depression as other anti-arrhythmic drugs. It can be used for both supraventricular and ventricular arrhythmias. It has many potential toxic effects.

Absolute contraindications. These include: sinus node or sino-atrial disease; pregnancy and breast feeding; (for i.v. use) severe respiratory failure; severe hypotension; severe cardiac failure; thyroid dysfunction; iodine sensitivity.

Relative contraindications. These include: renal impairment; cardiac failure; old age.

Side-effects. These are numerous and sometimes serious. They include: peripheral neuropathy; myopathy; bradycardia; potentiation of the effects of digoxin (which should be stopped or reduced when amiodarone is being given); phototoxicity; hypo- or hyperthyroidism; pulmonary alveolitis; hepatitis; headache.

Dose. Oral: 200 mg 3 times daily for a week, then 200 mg twice daily for a week, then 100–200 mg daily
i.v.: 1200 mg by infusion over 24 hours. The initial dose is usually 5 mg/kg, given over 30 min, followed by the remainder of the 1200 mg over the succeeding 23½ hours.

Amiodarone infusion must always be given via a central venous catheter.

Mexiletine

This drug is similar in its actions to lignocaine and can also be given by mouth. Effective dosing is often limited by side-effects, especially nausea and vomiting.

Absolute contraindication. Heart block.

Relative contraindication. Hepatic impairment.

Side-effects. These include: hypotension; bradycardia; confusion; convulsions; nausea and vomiting; psychiatric disturbances; nystagmus; tremor, jaundice.

Dose. Oral: 400 mg initially, then 200 mg 2 hours later, then 200–250 mg 3 to 4 times daily

i.v. : 100–250 mg at a rate of 25 mg per minute, then by infusion of 250 mg as 0.1% solution over 1 hour, then 250 mg over 2 hours then 0.5 mg/min.

Propafenone

This is a new drug which is still being evaluated. It has some beta-blocking activity.

Absolute contraindications. These include: obstructive airways disease; congestive heart failure; cardiogenic shock; severe bradycardia; sinus node disease; myasthenia gravis; second- or third-degree AV block or bundle branch block (BBB).

Relative contraindications. These include: hepatic or renal impairment; old age; the elderly; pregnancy.

Side-effects. These include: constipation; blurred vision; dry mouth; dizziness; nausea and vomiting; fatigue; diarrhoea; headache; allergic skin reactions.

Dose. Adults: 150 mg 3 times daily, increased after 3 days to 300 mg twice daily and then 300 mg 3 times daily if needed.

Lower doses in the elderly and in patients weighing less than 70 kg.

DRUGS ACTING ON THE CENTRAL NERVOUS SYSTEM (CNS)

HYPNOTICS

These drugs are still over-used and alternatives to hypnotics should be considered, such as a dose of analgesic at bed-time. Their use is, however, justified in some patients who are anxious about being in hospital. There is a danger of dependence so prescription should be limited to a week.

BENZODIAZEPINES

Temazepam, loprazolam and lormetazepam are short-acting, nitrazepam, flurazepam and diazepam are longer-acting, with a consequently greater risk of drowsiness.

Absolute contraindications. These include : respiratory depression; severe lung disease; phobic or obsessional states.

Relative contraindications. These include: chronic lung disease; personality disorders; muscle weakness; pregnancy and breast feeding; old age; hepatic or renal disease.

Side-effects. These include: drowsiness and light-headedness the next day; confusion; dependence.

Dose. Temazepam: 10–30 mg at night (elderly 5–15 mg)
Loprazolam: 1–2 mg at night (elderly 0.5–1 mg)
Lormetazepam: 0.5–1.5 mg at night (elderly 0.5 mg)
Nitrazepam: 5–10 mg at night (elderly 2.5–5 mg)
Diazepam: 5–15 mg at night.

CHLORAL

The only drug in this group which is commonly used in adults is chloral betaine (Welldorm); it is said to cause less respiratory depression than benzodiazepines.

Absolute contraindications. These include: severe cardiac disease; gastritis; marked liver or renal impairment.

Relative contraindications. These include: respiratory disease; severe personality disorder; pregnancy or breast feeding; old age.

Side-effects. These include: drowsiness the next day; gastric irritation; flatulence; rashes.

Dose. Adults: 1–2 tablets, with water, at night or 15–45 ml of elixir, with water, at night.

CHLORMETHIAZOLE

This causes less hangover than other drugs and may sometimes, therefore, be useful in the elderly. It is absolutely contraindicated in respiratory failure.

Relative contraindications. These include: cardiac and respiratory disease; a history of drug abuse; personality disorder; pregnancy and breast feeding; liver or renal impairment.

Side-effects. These include: nasal irritation and congestion; conjunctival irritation; headache; gastrointestinal disturbances.

Dose. Adults: 1–2 capsules or 5–10 ml syrup at bed-time.

ZOPICLONE

This is a relatively new drug. It is said to have a lower potential for dependence and abuse than benzodiazepines, though this remains to be proven. There are no absolute contraindications to its use.

Relative contraindications. These include: liver disease; pregnancy and breast feeding; old age; a history of drug abuse; psychiatric illness.

Side effects. These include: abnormal taste; GI disturbances; drowsiness the next day; irritability; confusion; depressed mood.

Dose. Adults: 7.5–15 mg at bed-time; elderly 3.75 mg.

ANTICONVULSANTS (→ also p 107)

For the emergency treatment of a fit, give Diazemuls, 10–20 mg intravenously *slowly* (5 mg per minute) or 10 mg of diazepam rectally. If fits recur after two doses of i.v. or rectal diazepam you should start the patient on an infusion of phenytoin (→ p 109).

For maintenance treatment of epilepsy, single anticonvulsants are to be preferred wherever possible. The choice of drug should normally be made by a more senior member of your team.

CARBAMAZEPINE

This is useful in a wide variety of different forms of epilepsy.

Absolute contraindications. These include various forms of AV conduction disorders.

Relative contraindications. These include hepatic impairment.

Side-effects. These are common, especially with higher doses. They include : GI disturbances; dizziness; drowsiness; headache; ataxia; confusion; constipation; anorexia; generalized rash.

Dose. Adults: 100–200 mg twice daily, increased gradually to between 800 mg and 1.2 g daily in divided doses.

> ➘ Plasma levels, taken together with clinical effects, can provide guidance as to dosage requirement. Therapeutic range 4–12 mg/litre (20–50 μmol/l).

PHENYTOIN

This drug is widely used for both tonic-clonic and partial epilepsy. There are no absolute contraindications but side-effects are common and the drug has a narrow therapeutic window (i.e. the effective dose is close to the toxic dose). Small increases in dosage can result in large increases in blood levels.

Relative contraindications. These include: liver disease; pregnancy.

Side-effects. These include: nausea and vomiting; confusion; dizziness; tremor; nystagmus; ataxia; rashes; facial coarsening; hirsutism; megaloblastic anaemia.

Dose. Adults: oral — 150–300 mg daily initially, increased to 400–600 mg per day if needed; doses higher than 300 mg per day should be divided in two.
i.v. — (→ p 109).

> ➘ Blood levels are very helpful in adjusting the dose of phenytoin, though clinical effect must also be considered. Therapeutic range 10–20 mg/l (40–80 μmol/l).

SODIUM VALPROATE

This is a very useful drug for tonic-clonic seizures and is the drug of choice for myoclonic epilepsy.

Absolute contraindications. These include: moderate or severe liver disease; possibility of pregnancy or pregnant state up to 13 weeks' gestation (high risk of neural tube defects).

Relative contraindications. These include a risk of significant liver disease.

Side-effects. These include: gastric irritation; nausea; tremor; weight gain; transient hair loss; oedema; thrombocytopenia and impaired platelet function; amenorrhoea.

Dose. Adults: 200 mg 3 times a day, increased gradually if necessary to between 1 g and 2 g daily; maximum 2.5 g daily.

> Blood levels of valproate, though easy to measure, are a poor guide to dosage requirement. The only value of measuring blood levels is to make sure that the patient is actually taking the tablets.

PHENOBARBITONE

This drug is useful for both tonic-clonic and partial seizures but often causes sedation. It is sometimes used in combination with another anticonvulsant in difficult cases. There are many possible interactions with other drugs.

Relative contraindications. These include: impaired liver or renal function; old age; respiratory depression (to be avoided if severe).

Side-effects. These include: drowsiness; lethargy; depression; ataxia; allergic skin reactions; restlessness and confusion; megaloblastic anaemia.

Dose. Adults: oral — 60–180 mg at night
i.m. — 50–200 mg repeated after 6 hours if necessary.

LAMOTRIGINE AND VIGABATRIN

These are very new drugs which appear to have great potential in patients with difficult epilepsy. They should not be used except in specialist neurological units.

DRUGS FOR PARKINSONISM

LEVODOPA

This is the drug of choice for patients with disability due to idiopathic Parkinson's disease. It is less valuable in older than in younger patients and in those with long-standing disease. It is best given with a peripheral decarboxylase inhibitor so as to reduce the incidence of non-CNS side-effects. Low doses should be used initially and dose increases should be gradual. It should not be used in drug-induced Parkinsonism.

Contraindications. Glaucoma.

Relative contraindications. These include: lung disease; peptic ulceration; cardiovascular disease; psychiatric illness.

Side-effects. These include: anorexia; nausea and vomiting; agitation; postural hypotension; dizziness; involuntary movements; hypomania or psychosis.

Dose. Sinemet Plus — 1 tablet 3 times daily, increased gradually. Higher doses may be given as Sinemet or Sinemet CR instead of Sinemet Plus.

Madopar 62.5 — 1 capsule twice daily (for heavier patients, start with Madopar 125). Higher doses may be given as Madopar 250 or Madopar CR.

BROMOCRIPTINE

This drug acts as a dopamine agonist but has few advantages over levodopa. You should not initiate treatment with bromocriptine except with the advice of a senior colleague.

SELEGILINE

This drug is helpful, as an adjunct to levodopa, in patients with end-of-dose deterioration in symptoms. Some neurologists also believe that it slows the progression of Parkinson's disease, though this remains unproven. Selegiline interacts with levodopa, the dosage of which may need to be reduced by 20-50% when selegiline is added.

Side-effects. These include: hypotension; nausea and vomiting; confusion; agitation.

Dose. 10 mg daily, in the morning, or 5 mg at breakfast and at mid-day.

LYSURIDE AND PERGOLIDE

These are recently introduced dopamine agonists whose place in treatment is not fully defined. They should not be used outside specialist units.

ANTIMUSCARINIC DRUGS

These are weaker than levodopa but are useful for patients with milder symptoms, especially tremor and rigidity. They are also of value in the treatment of drug-induced Parkinsonism and can be given by injection.

Benzhexol, orphenadrine and procyclidine

These are the most widely used drugs.

Absolute contraindications. These include: urinary retention; closed-angle glaucoma; GI obstruction.

Relative contraindications. These include: cardiovascular disease; hepatic or renal impairment.

Side-effects. These include: dry mouth; blurred vision; dizziness; GI disturbances; urinary retention; nervousness; confusion; psychiatric disturbances.

Dose. Oral:

benzhexol	—	1 mg daily, increased gradually to 5–15 mg/day in 3–4 doses
orphenadrine	—	150 mg daily in divided doses, gradually increased; maximum 400 mg/day
procyclidine	—	2.5 mg 3 times a day, gradually increased; maximum 30 mg/day.
i.m. : procyclidine	—	5–10 mg, repeated if necessary after 20 min; maximum 20 mg/day
i.v. : procyclidine	—	5 mg (usually effective within 5 min), occasionally 10 mg needed.

Benztropine

This is similar to benzhexol but it tends to cause sedation rather than stimulation. It can be given by injection.

Dose. Oral : 0.5–1 mg daily at bed–time, increased gradually to 1–4 mg daily; maximum 6 mg daily

i.m. or i.v.: 1–2 mg, repeated if symptoms recur.

DRUGS ACTING ON THE GASTROINTESTINAL (GI) TRACT

INDIGESTION

Symptomatic remedies are undoubtedly valuable for short-term use and in this context simple antacids should be used first: do not go straight to more powerful drugs such as H_2-receptor antagonists. If symptoms persist, further investigation by endoscopy or X-ray studies is usually necessary. There are many preparations on the market, so try to become familiar with just two or three of them.

ANTACIDS

Magnesium trisilicate mixture

This is widely used and generally well-tolerated. It should be used with caution or avoided in those at risk of cardiac, hepatic or renal failure as it contains significant amounts of sodium (6 mmol/10 ml). It can cause diarrhoea.

Dose. 10 mg 3 times daily.

Co-magaldrox (Maalox)

This is a suitable alternative to magnesium trisilicate. It is very low in sodium and is widely prescribed as a tablet for those who prefer it. Maalox is more expensive than magnesium trisilicate.

Dose. Tablets: 1–2 tablets, chewed, 20 minutes after meals and at bed-time

Suspension: 5–10 ml 3–4 times daily as required (usually after meals and at bed-time).

Alginate-containing antacids

These are preferred by some patients, particularly those with reflux oesophagitis. Gastrocote and Gaviscon are the most widely prescribed brands; Gastrocote is slightly lower in sodium than Gaviscon.

Dose. Tablets: 1–2 tablets up to 4 times daily

Liquid: 5–20 ml 4 times daily.

In either case the preparation is usually given after meals and at bed-time.

H_2-RECEPTOR ANTAGONISTS

These drugs are useful in the treatment of peptic ulceration and in reflux oesophagitis. They also promote healing in ulceration associated with NSAIDs. There is no evidence that newer (and more expensive) drugs are better than older ones. There is no good evidence that H_2-receptor antagonists are of value in the treatment of acute GI haemorrhage and it is, therefore, *rarely (if ever) necessary* to give them by injection.

Cimetidine

This is the best-known and cheapest H_2-receptor antagonist available.

Relative contraindications. These include: renal and hepatic impairment; pregnancy and breast feeding; old age.

Side-effects. These are rare but include: dizziness; altered bowel habit; confusion (especially in the elderly); gynaecomastia. There are also significant drug interactions with warfarin, phenytoin and theophyllines.

Dose. 400 mg twice daily or 800 mg at night.

Ranitidine

This is more expensive than cimetidine but has fewer side-effects and does not interact with other drugs. It is probably more suitable for the elderly because it is less likely to cause confusion.

Dose. 150–300 mg twice a day or 300 mg at night.

OMEPRAZOLE

This drug is a powerful inhibitor of gastric acid secretion. Its main use is in the treatment of severe, ulcerative oesophagitis. It should not be used in patients who have not been investigated.

Absolute contraindications. These include pregnancy and breast feeding.

Relative contraindications. These include severe liver disease.

Side-effects. These include: diarrhoea; headache; nausea; constipation; dizziness; somnolence; skin reactions; photosensitivity; muscle and joint pain; oedema.

Dose. 20 mg daily for 4 weeks; in severe cases 40 mg daily for up to 8 weeks.

BISMUTH

This drug is the treatment of choice for gastritis or duodenitis associated with *Heliocobacter pylori* infection. To be fully effective the drug must be given in combination with antibiotics.

Contraindications. Bismuth chelate is contraindicated in severe renal impairment.

Side-effects. The drug causes blackening of the stools (warn the patient) and may blacken the tongue. Nausea and vomiting may also occur.

Dose. As De-Noltab: 2 tablets twice a day for 4 weeks. For the first 2 weeks, give metronidazole 400 mg 8 hourly plus either amoxycillin 250 mg 8 hourly or tetracycline 250 mg 6 hourly.

LAXATIVES

These drugs should only be used if you are satisfied that the patient has true constipation (not just infrequent bowel actions) and after intestinal obstruction has been excluded.

BULK LAXATIVES

These should be taken with adequate fluid.

Side-effects. These are rare except for nausea, which may limit their use. Some patients also report troublesome flatulence.

Dose. Adults: Trifyba — 1 sachet, added to food, 2–3 times daily
Fybogel — half — 1 sachet once or twice daily
Regulan — half —1 sachet once or twice daily.

OSMOTIC LAXATIVES

These are effective and safe but frequently produce diarrhoea if given in large doses or for too long.

Dose. Lactulose: 15 ml twice daily, reduced as needed.

STIMULANT LAXATIVES

Senna

This is generally safe if used appropriately. It is very economical.

Dose. Adults: 2–4 tablets at night.

Docusate sodium (Dioctyl)

This is preferred by some physicians and can be given either as a tablet or a liquid.

Dose. Adults: up to 5 tablets or 50 ml of solution daily, in divided doses.

Co-danthramer and Co-danthrusate

These are frowned upon because of a possible risk of carcinogenesis (suggested by animal studies). They are, however, popular with the elderly and are also useful in terminal care, as an adjunct to potent analgesics.

Side-effects. These include red discoloration of the urine (warn the patient) and skin irritation (in the incontinent).

Dose. Adults: 1–3 capsules or 5–10 ml of suspension at bedtime.

RECTAL PREPARATIONS

Glycerine suppositories

These are useful in patients who are constipated for some short-term reason such as immobilization.

Enemas

These are of use in patients with constipation or faecal impaction who cannot swallow. Sodium citrate enemas (e.g. Micralax) or phosphate enemas (e.g. Fletchers' Phosphate Enema) are milder; arachis oil enemas are more potent and are more effective as stool softeners.

DRUGS FOR NAUSEA AND VOMITING

(→ also pp 68–69)

PROCHLORPERAZINE

This is a good anti-emetic which can be given both orally and by injection. It has many potential side-effects.

Absolute contraindications. These are few but include bone-marrow depression.

Relative contraindications. These include: cardiovascular disease; epilepsy (lowers the fit threshold); pregnancy and breast feeding; parkinsonism; renal and hepatic disease; a history of jaundice.

Side-effects. These include: involuntary movements (especially in children and young adults); extrapyramidal symptoms; dry mouth; hypothermia; hypotension; alteration in liver function (including frank jaundice).

Dose. Adults: oral — 20 mg initially, then 10 mg after 2 hours. For prophylaxis 5–10 mg 2–3 times daily
buccal — 1–2 tablets twice daily, inserted between the gum and upper lip
rectal — 25 mg, followed if necessary by 10–20 mg 6 hours later
i.m. (deep) or i.v. — 12.5 mg up to 4 hourly.

METOCLOPRAMIDE

This is again a very effective drug. There is, however, a high incidence of dystonic reactions in young people, so this drug should **not be given to those under 20** except with specialist advice.

Relative contraindications. These include: hepatic and renal impairment; pregnancy (though the dangers of this have probably been overstated); recent GI surgery (best avoided).

Side-effects. These include: dystonic and other extrapyramidal reactions; drowsiness; diarrhoea.

Dose. Adults: oral, i.m. or i.v. — 10 mg up to 4 times daily
chemotherapy — by continuous i.v. infusion, 2–4 mg per kg over 15–30 min then 3–5 mg per kg over 8–12 hours (maximum over 24 h 10 mg per kg).

DOMPERIDONE

This drug does not cross the blood-brain barrier except in small amounts so it is unsuitable for the treatment of nausea due to vestibular or CNS disease. It is particularly useful if the nausea is due to oesophageal or gastric causes, including reflux. It cannot be given by injection.

Relative contraindications. These include: pregnancy and breast feeding. Not recommended for chronic administration.

Side-effects. These are uncommon but acute dystonic reactions are reported.

Dose. Adults: oral – 10–20 mg every 4–8 hours
rectal – 30–60 mg every 4–8 hours.

CISAPRIDE

This is not strictly an anti-emetic, rather it enhances peristalsis and increased tone in the lower oesophageal sphincter. It is particularly useful for patients with persistent vomiting due to a hiatus hernia or to oesophageal dysmotility (e.g. diabetic autonomic neuropathy).

Contraindications. Pregnancy.

Relative contraindications. These include : hepatic and renal impairment; old age.

Side-effects. These include: abdominal cramps; diarrhoea; headaches.

Dose. Adults: oral — 10 mg 3–4 times daily, usually for 6–12 weeks.
Maintenance treatment : 20 mg at bed-time.

ONDANSETRON AND GRANISETRON

These drugs are used for the prevention and treatment of vomiting associated with chemotherapy for malignant disease. They may in certain circumstances, be combined with dexamethasone. For dosage schedules, consult a senior member of your team or the BNF.

ANTIDIARRHOEAL AGENTS (→ also pp 77–80)

It is usually unnecessary to treat diarrhoea specifically, as it is often self-limiting. If diarrhoea is due to infection the use of anti-diarrhoeal drugs will prolong it. Where symptomatic treatment is required, use loperamide or codeine phosphate.

CODEINE PHOSPHATE

This drug is generally safe in adults, but should not be given to children. It should be used cautiously in renal impairment.

Side-effects. The commonest, not surprisingly, is constipation. Nausea and vomiting are a problem for some patients.

Dose. Oral: 30–60 mg 3– 4 times daily.

LOPERAMIDE

This drug has similar properties to codeine (→ above) but is a little more powerful. It may cause abdominal cramps and skin reactions.

Dose. Adults: 4 mg initially then 2 mg after each loose stool for up to 5 days. Usual dose 6–8 mg per day, maximum 16 mg per day.

DRUGS FOR CHEST DISEASES

BRONCHODILATORS

BETA-ADRENERGIC AGONISTS

The treatment of acute asthma depends crucially on the use of nebulized beta-adrenergic agonists, chiefly salbutamol and terbutaline (→ pp 225–226). If you are treating asthma the nebulizer should be driven by *oxygen*; if, however, the patient has chronic bronchitis or any past history of carbon dioxide retention, it should be driven by *air*.

Salbutamol

This drug is extremely effective and usually well-tolerated.

Side-effects. The commonest is tremor if the drug is given in large doses. It should be used with caution in patients with hyperthyroidism or severe ischaemic heart disease or a history of cardiac arrhythmias.

> **If you are giving intravenous salbutamol to a patient with diabetes, monitor the blood glucose carefully; loss of diabetic control, and even ketoacidosis, have been reported.**

Other side-effects include: headache; palpitations; hypokalaemia (which can be severe). Nebulized salbutamol should be mixed in normal saline, not water.

> Remember to monitor the serum potassium closely when treating severe asthma.

Dose. By nebulizer: 2.5–5 mg every 4–6 hours
i.v.: 5 μg per minute initially, adjusted as necessary within the range 3–20 μg/min.

Once the patient is well enough not to need salbutamol by nebulizer it can be given by inhaler. A metered-dose aerosol is effective if used properly but fails in many cases because the patient cannot coordinate breathing with pressing the inhaler button; in such cases a volume spacer (Volumatic) may be helpful. Alternatively, a different form of inhaler may be suitable such as a breath-actuated device (Aerolin Auto-haler) or a dry powder device (Ventolin Rota-haler).

Metered dose inhaler: 100–200 μg 3–4 times daily
Dry powder inhaler: 200–400 μg 3–4 times daily.

> If a patient is having problems using inhalers, ask the pharmacist or physiotherapist to display a range of inhalers so that a choice can be made.

Tablets: 8–16 mg every 12 hours. Oral salbutamol is of little value but some patients with chronic bronchitis like it, particularly to help them with sleep.

Terbutaline

This is very similar in its properties and usage to salbutamol. Some patients prefer the dry powder form of this drug (Bricanyl Turbo-haler) to the corresponding form of salbutamol.

Dose. Nebulizer: 5–10 mg every 4–6 hours
i.v.: 2–5 μg per minute (occasionally more for short periods)
Inhaler: 500 μg 2–4 times daily.

Salmeterol

This drug is longer acting than salbutamol or terbutaline and is used in patients who have troublesome or 'difficult' asthma. Such patients should also be taking an inhaled steroid or cromoglycate. Salmeterol should *not* be used for the immediate relief of acute attacks of bronchospasm.

Side-effects. These are similar to those of salbutamol. There is a significant incidence of paradoxical bronchoconstriction with this drug.

Dose. Inhaler: 50–100 μg every 12 hours.

ANTIMUSCARINIC DRUGS

These drugs may be a useful adjunct to treatment with beta-agonists, particularly in patients with chronic bronchitis.

Ipratropium bromide (Atrovent)

This drug is relatively safe with few serious side-effects, though dry mouth occurs occasionally. High doses are potentially risky in patients with glaucoma.

Dose. Nebulizer: 200–500 μg 4 times daily
Inhaler: 20–80 μg 3–4 times daily.

THEOPHYLLINES

These drugs provide relief of bronchial constriction and may be useful in both asthma and chronic bronchitis, particularly the latter. They may have an additive effect when combined with beta-agonists. They have a narrow margin between therapeutic and toxic dose and there are differences in bioavailability between brands, so it is now recommended that prescribers should specify which brand of theophylline is to be used.

Theophyllines should be used with *caution* in patients with heart failure, epilepsy or cirrhosis and in the elderly.

Side-effects. These include: nausea; tachycardia; palpitations; headache; convulsions; cardiac arrhythmias (including ventricular fibrillation); hypokalaemia.

Theophyllines display a number of important interactions with other drugs: the half-life is *increased* by ciprofloxacin, erythromycin, cimetidine and oral contraceptives; it is *decreased* by smoking and heavy drinking and by enzyme-inducing drugs such as phenytoin, carbamazepine, rifampicin and barbiturates.

Safe use of theophyllines is greatly enhanced by *monitoring of plasma levels*, which should be maintained within the range 10–20 mg/l (55–110 μmol/l).

Dose.	Oral:	Nuelin SA	— 175–500 mg every 12 hours
		Slo-Phyllin	— 250–500 mg every 12 hours
		Phyllocontin	— 225–450 mg every 12 hours
		Theo-Dur	— 200 mg every 12 hours
		Uniphyllin	— 200–400 mg every 12 hours.

It may be appropriate to give a larger dose of theophylline in the evening than in the morning in order to relieve symptoms of nocturnal bronchospasm.

Intravenous aminophylline

This may be given by very slow bolus injection but you should not do this without advice and instruction from your SHO or registrar. For advice on the use of aminophylline by infusion, → p 226.

INHALED STEROIDS

Any patient with asthma, or chronic bronchitis with some reversibility, must be thought of as a potential candidate for inhaled corticosteroids; the only exception would be someone with very mild asthma whose symptoms are easily controlled with inhaled beta-adrenergic agonists needed infrequently.

It is *essential* that patients understand that inhaled steroids do not relieve acute breathlessness and that they must be used continuously.

Side-effects. These are few, but if used in high doses they can show effects similar to those of oral steroids, notably bone thinning and adrenal suppression. Inhaled steroids may also cause sore throat and oropharyngeal thrush.

As with beta-adrenergic agonists, inhaled steroids will only provide benefit if used correctly. Metered-dose aerosols are unsuitable for many patients because they cannot coordinate breathing with pressing the inhaler button; in such cases a volume spacer (Volumatic or Nebu-haler) may be helpful. Alternatively one can use a different form of inhaler such as a breath-actuated device (AeroBec Autohaler) or a dry powder inhaler (Becotide Rota-haler, Pulmicort Turbo-haler). Steroids may also be given by nebulizer.

Dose.			
	Inhaler	Becotide Aerobec	100–200 μg 3– 4 times daily or 200–400 μg twice daily
	Dry powder inhaler	Becotide Rotacaps	200 μg 3–4 times daily or 400 μg twice daily
	High-dose inhaler	Becloforte AeroBec Forte	500 μg twice daily or 250 μg 4 times daily
	Dry powder inhaler	Pulmicort Turbo-haler	200 μg twice daily
	Nebulizer	Pulmicort Respules	1–2 mg twice daily, diluted if necessary with 0.9% saline.

SODIUM CROMOGLYCATE

This drug can reduce the incidence of attacks of asthma, particularly in children and young adults. It is also useful for the prophylaxis of exercise-induced asthma, being taken half an hour before exercise. Some patients find the dry powder form causes bronchospasm, in which case a beta-agonist inhaler should be used a few minutes before the cromoglycate. It is *essential* that patients understand that cromoglycate is of no value in relieving acute bronchospasm and that it only works if taken continuously. The use of compound inhalers which contain isoprenaline and cromoglycate (Intal Co) is not recommended as neither drug is being used to optimal effect.

Dose. Inhaler: 10 mg 4 times daily, increased in severe cases to 6–8 times daily

Dry powder inhaler: 20 mg 4 times daily, increased in severe cases to 8 times daily

Nebulized: 20 mg 4 times daily, increased if needed to 6 times daily.

> It is difficult to predict which patients with asthma will respond to cromoglycate. A 4-week trial is reasonable: if the patient has shown no response in this time, cromoglycate should be stopped and an inhaled corticosteroid considered instead.

OXYGEN

Oxygen should be regarded as a drug and should be prescibed on the routine prescription sheet. It can be given either by face mask or nasal cannulae. Patients' reactions to oxygen administration vary: some find it comforting and seem to get as much psychological as physiological benefit from it, while others find the face mask claustrophobic. On the whole it is unwise to use oxygen as a placebo.

The aim of oxygen therapy should be to maintain the patient's arterial PO_2 within the range 10–14 kPa (75–105 mmHg). The amount of oxygen delivered to the patient depends on the type of mask used and the flow rate: many hospitals use a range of masks or mask adaptors which contain a venturi type of delivery system (e.g. Venti-mask); these are often colour–coded. Make sure that you understand which mask is which and what flow rate is recommended (→ Table 4.3)

Table 4.3
Flow rates for oxygen delivery ('Lifecare' mask system)

24% – 2 l/min
28% – 4 l/min
35% – 8 l/min
40% – 8 l/min
60% – 12 l/min

Oxygen concentration. For primary hypoxic illnesses such as pneumonia, pulmonary embolism, pulmonary fibrosis and also for acute LVF, give the highest flow rate that the patient can comfortably tolerate, i.e., 40% or more. If a bed-side pulse oximeter is available, aim to keep the saturation level above 90%. After an hour or so, re-check the blood gases to ensure that the PaO_2 is within the required range. High concentrations of oxygen (60%) should not be used for long periods without the advice of a more senior member of the firm.

In chronic bronchitis, give 28% oxygen initially, then re-check the blood gases after half an hour to make sure that the PaO_2 is not rising. You may need to reduce the oxygen concentration to 24% or even discontinue it (→ below).

In asthma, give 60% oxygen initially. However, it is particularly important to watch out for CO_2 retention, so *be sure to recheck the blood gases* 1 to 2 hours after starting oxygen.

> **If you cannot maintain the PaO_2 above 8 k*Pa* then the patient is in respiratory failure and may need respiratory stimulants or mechanical ventilation: consult your SHO or registrar.**
> **If the $Paco_2$ rises above 8.0 k*Pa* (6.0 k*Pa* in the case of acute asthma) the situation is again one of respiratory failure and is potentially dangerous. The patient may need respiratory stimulants or mechanical ventilation: consult your SHO or registrar.**

DOXAPRAM

This drug is a respiratory stimulant which acts on the respiratory centre. It is not a substitute for bronchodilators, antibiotics, chest physiotherapy, etc. but can be a useful adjunct to these measures in getting people, particularly those with chronic chest disease, over a crisis without the need for mechanical ventilation.

Contraindications. These include: severe hypertension; coronary artery disease; thyrotoxicosis.

Relative contraindications. These include: epilepsy; liver disease.

Dose. i.v. infusion: 1.5–4 mg per minute, adjusted according to the results of blood gas measurements.

CORTICOSTEROIDS

Steroids have a wide variety of uses. As a house physician you are most likely to be asked to prescribe them for asthma, inflammatory bowel disease, rheumatic diseases (mainly polymyalgia rheumatica and SLE), cerebral oedema or, occasionally, for people with adrenal insufficiency.

> **Steroids are of no value in patients with septicaemia, even if shocked. Their role in rheumatoid arthritis is very limited, being confined essentially to intra-articular injection. You should not prescribe systemic steroids in rheumatoid arthritis except under the supervision of a specialist rheumatologist.**

Prednisolone

This is the most widely used systemic steroid. It is very potent but has many potential side-effects.

Contraindications. There are none.

Relative contraindications. These include: diabetes mellitus; peptic ulceration; osteoporosis; psychiatric disease; undiagnosed fever.

Side-effects. These include : glucose intolerance (provoking latent diabetes or worsening the control of existing diabetes); mental disturbances including euphoria, paranoid psychosis; dyspepsia or peptic ulceration; suppression of signs of infection (allowing it to spread unnoticed). In long-term use steroids can cause osteoporosis; avascular necrosis of the femoral head; skin atrophy; muscle wasting; adrenal suppression; Cushing's syndrome.

> **Patients taking steroids for more than a few weeks should carry a steroid card; these are obtainable from hospital pharmacies or Family Health Services Authorities (FHSAs).**

Side-effects are unlikely if the dose of prednisolone is less than 7 mg per day, though there is still a possibility of adrenal suppression. Adverse effects are further reduced if maintenance prednisolone is given on alternate days rather than daily. Where possible, prednisolone should be given once daily in the morning; it is only necessary to divide up the dose if this makes tablet taking more convenient.

Dose. Adults:

asthma	— 30–40 mg per day
polymyalgia rheumatica	— 10–20 mg per day
cranial arteritis	— 40–60 mg per day
inflammatory bowel disease	— 20–40 mg per day orally or 60–80 mg per day i.v.
SLE	— 30–60 mg per day
polymyositis	— 1–2mg/kg per day.

Dexamethasone

This is the steroid of choice for the treatment of cerebral oedema. Its side-effects are the same as those of prednisolone; however, it is rarely necessary to give dexamethasone long-term.

Dose. Adults:

oral —	4 mg 6 hourly, reduced after a few days to 2–4 mg 3 times daily
i.m. —	10 mg initially, then 4 mg 4 times a day
i.v. —	(slow injection or infusion) 10 mg initially, then 4 mg 4 times a day.

Hydrocortisone

This is the compound of choice for steroid replacement in people with adrenal insufficiency or hypopituitarism. It is also used for urgent treatment in asthma, inflammatory bowel disease, etc. and in patients with adrenal insufficiency who cannot take their treatment orally. Hydrocortisone has mineralocorticoid activity and is more likely than other steroids to cause fluid retention and hypertension. Side-effects do *not* occur when hydrocortisone is given in appropriate replacement doses; if side-effects are, apparently, occurring then the 'replacement' dose being given is too high.

Dose.

Oral, for adrenal replacement:	10–20 mg on waking, plus 5–10 mg at tea-time; occasional patients also require 5–10 mg at lunch-time
i.m. or i.v.:	100–200 mg every 6 hours.

Patients on long-term steroids who develop any intercurrent illness (infection, fracture, MI, etc.) should have the steroid dose increased to *at least double the normal* amount during the acute phase of the illness. In patients who cannot swallow, hydrocortisone should be given by injection in a dose of 100-200 mg 3–4 times daily.

ANTICOAGULANTS

Heparin

Heparin is usually given i.v. and secures rapid anticoagulation. Its effect cannot be predicted and laboratory monitoring by means of the activated partial thromboplastin time (APTT), or a similar test, is essential.

Side-effects. Other than bleeding these are unlikely to be troublesome in short-term use; however, a small percentage of patients given heparin for more than 7 days will develop thrombocytopenia.

Contraindications. Use in those with a known bleeding disorder and in anyone who has had a recent operation on the eye or the CNS or who has had a recent stroke, unless a CT scan has shown it to be non-haemorrhagic.

Dose. It is also possible to give heparin subcutaneously as calcium heparin, 17500 iu 12 hourly. Although subcutaneous heparin is probably as effective as the i.v. form it is not widely used in the UK for therapeutic, as distinct from prophylactic, purposes. It is wise, therefore, to consult a senior member of your firm if you are considering using s.c. heparin therapeutically.

The initial loading dose is 5000 iu, given as an intravenous bolus. The loading dose should be reduced for children and for small adults. Follow this up with an i.v. infusion of heparin, diluted in saline, starting at 1400 iu/hour.

Dosage adjustment. The APTT should be measured 6 hours after the start of the infusion and the infusion rate adjusted according to the guidelines given in Table 4.4.

Table 4.4
Heparin infusion schedule*

Loading dose	5000 iu i.v. over 5 minutes
Initial infusion rate	25000 iu heparin made up in saline to 50 ml gives a final concentration of 500 iu/ml, to be started at 2.8 ml/hr (1400 iu/hr)

Check APTT at 6 hours. Adjust according to APTT ratio (APTT: control) as follows:

APTT ratio	Infusion rate change
> 7	Stop for 30 min to 1 hour and reduce by 500 iu/h
5.1–7.0	Reduce by 500 iu/h
4.1–5.0	Reduce by 300 iu/h
3.1–4.0	Reduce by 100 iu/h
2.6–3.0	Reduce by 50 iu/h
1.5–2.5	No change
1.2–1.4	Increase by 200 iu/h
<1.2	Increase by 400 iu/h

After each change wait 10 hours before next APTT estimation unless APTT ratio is > 5.0, when estimates should be made more frequently, e.g. 4-hourly.

* Suggested heparin schedule based on APTT measurement. Modified from Fennerty et al. *British Medical Journal* 1988; 297: 1285–8.

After a dosage change the APTT should be measured again 10 or more hours later and further adjustments made if necessary. Once a stable state is reached, measure the APTT daily.

> Blood samples for APTT must reach the laboratory within 1 hour of being taken if the result is to be accurate. Do not leave the sample in the ward fridge for a porter's round several hours later.

Duration of treatment. For most patients with DVT or pulmonary embolism which are not massive, 5 days' treatment with heparin, with warfarin started on day 1, are sufficient. Longer treatment may be needed for major pulmonary embolism or iliofemoral DVT. Consult a senior member of your firm.

Treatment of haemorrhage. It is usually sufficient to stop the heparin, as it has a very short half-life. For severe bleeding protamine sulphate, a specific antidote, should be given in a dose of 1 mg for every 100 iu of heparin infused over the previous hour. The dose of protamine should be halved if the heparin has been stopped for 1 hour and reduced to a quarter if stopped for 2 hours. Remember to check the APTT again 2–4 hours after giving protamine: it is cleared from the circulation more rapidly than heparin so a repeat dose may have to be given.

Prophylactic heparin

Prophylactic heparin, given subcutaneously, is indicated not just for surgical patients but for a variety of bed-bound medical patients who, by reason of a serious disease, are at increased risk of DVT (Table 4.5). The usual dose is 5000 iu given every 9–12 hours. Laboratory monitoring is not required except in pregnancy, when a senior physician or clinical haematologist should be involved in the treatment. Prophylactic anticoagulation can also be undertaken using various low-molecular-weight heparins (e.g. enoxaparin, dalteparin): these need to be given only once daily but their place in routine management is not yet established.

Table 4.5 Groups of bed-bound patients who should be considered for prophylactic s.c. heparin
Acute MI
Malignant disease
Stroke (non-haemorrhagic)
Respiratory failure
Congestive cardiac failure
IBD
Previous history of DVT/PE
Paraproteinaemia.

Side-effects. These become important if it is used long-term: they include: thrombocytopenia; osteoporosis; alopecia.

Warfarin

Warfarin is the drug of choice for long-term anticoagulation. It should be started at the same time as heparin, though in the case of massive iliofemoral thrombosis or PE, some authorities recommend starting warfarin on day 3. Warfarin is usually given at 5–7 p.m. and the INR measured the following morning.

Warfarin should not be given in pregnancy or in the presence of severe hypertension or infective endocarditis. It is not generally used in cerebral thrombosis or peripheral arterial occlusion but may be of value in transient ischaemic attacks.

Side-effects. The most important is, of course, haemorrhage (→ below). Other side-effects include alopecia.

Management of haemorrhage. If the INR is > 4.5 but there is no haemorrhage, stop warfarin for 1–2 days and repeat the INR. For minor bleeding 1 mg of i.v. vitamin K will speed the fall in INR without making the patient refractory to warfarin. For major bleeding, give 5 mg of vitamin K i.v., together with clotting factor concentrate or (more commonly) FFP, 2 units. In severe overdosage the vitamin K and/or FFP may need to be repeated. Consult your local haematologist.

Dose. The INR should be measured before starting warfarin. If the INR is normal two 10-mg doses of warfarin should be given 24 hours apart. If the INR is elevated, give 5 mg warfarin, then adjust the dose as indicated in Table 4.6. Further adjustment to the dose of warfarin should be as indicated in Table 4.6.

Table 4.6
Warfarin schedule *

Day	INR(9-11 a.m.)	Warfarin dose (mg) given at 5–7 p.m.
1st	< 1.4	10
	< 1.8	10
2nd	1.8	1
	> 1.8	0.5
	< 2.0	10
	2.0–2.1	5
	2.2–2.3	4.5
	2.4–2.5	4
	2.6–2.7	3.5
3rd	2.8–2.9	3
	3.0–3.1	2.5
	3.2–3.3	2
	3.4	1.5
	3.5	1
	3.6–4.0	0.5
	.> 4.0	0
		Predicted maintenance dose:
	< 1.4	> 8
	1.4	8
	1.5	7.5
	1.6–1.7	7
	1.8	6.5
	1.9	6
	2.0–2.1	5.5
4th	2.2–2.3	5
	2.4–2.6	4.5
	2.7–3.0	4
	3.1–3.5	3.5
	3.6–4.0	3
	4.1–4.5	Miss out next day‘s dose then give 2 mg
	>4.5	Miss out 2 day’s doses then give 1 mg

APTT should be within or below therapeutic range (1.5–2.5 times control). If APTT is above this range the heparin effect on INR should be neutralized by adding protamine (0.4mg/ml plasma) to the sample.

* Suggested warfarin schedule based on INR. Modified from Fennerty et al. *British Medical Journal* 1988; 297: 1285–8.

The recommended therapeutic range for INR will depend on the condition for which anticoagulation is being given (→ Table 4.7).

Table 4.7
Recommended therapeutic ranges for INR in different conditions

1.4–2.8	Patients with AF without history of thromboembolism
2.0–2.5	Prophylaxis of DVT related to surgery in high-risk patients
2.0–3.0	Prophylaxis in orthopaedic surgery. Treatment of DVT and PE. Prevention of embolism in patients with mitral stenosis, atrial fibrillation with a previous history of embolism, tissue prosthetic heart valves, TIA
3.0–4.5	Recurrent DVT or pulmonary embolism. Mechanical prosthetic heart valves.

Once the dosage of warfarin is stable, the INR should be measured weekly. The patient should be followed up in an anticoagulant clinic and should be given the Department of Health anticoagulation booklet.

! Warfarin interacts with many other drugs, especially aspirin and alcohol. Patients must be warned about this.

SECTION 5

Management of common conditions

PRIORITIES AT A CARDIAC ARREST

Being present at a cardiac arrest is one of the most stressful parts of a junior doctor's job. It is essential to be well prepared by attending a course in cardio-pulmonary resuscitation. Many hospitals now run such courses for their staff, but if yours does not, try to find out from the CCU or A & E department who the hospital resuscitation officer is. If all else fails, ask a member of the cardiology staff or a senior anaesthetist to organize a teaching session for you and a few colleagues.

Diagnosis of cardiac arrest

This is relatively simple, relying on just two criteria:

- loss of consciousness
- absence of a central pulse (carotid or femoral).

The patient may not stop breathing immediately after the arrest. It is *not* sensible or necessary to auscultate the heart or do any other test if the two criteria are satisfied.

Actions at the scene of the arrest

The urgent priority is resuscitation by means of artifical ventilation and cardiac massage; it is not necessary at the beginning to do an ECG, make a diagnosis or give any drugs. Therefore the order of proceeding is:

- Establish the diagnosis. Remember to call to the patient and to shake him/her to be sure that he/she is really unconscious
- Get the patient on to a hard surface (ideally a firm bed, possibly with a board under the mattress. If the patient is in a soft bed and there is no board, lift him/her carefully onto the floor
- Put your fingers in the patient's mouth and remove false teeth, food debris, etc.
- If the arrest has been witnessed, consider a single sharp, precordial thump
- Begin resuscitation using cardiac massage and artificial ventilation; ventilation by mouth-to-mouth means will do but a Brook airway is better and a face mask combined with an Ambu-bag is better still. *Do not* attempt to intubate the patient unless you are confident about this procedure
- If you are the only doctor at the arrest, do not attempt to do anything else until help arrives. Continue with cardiopulmonary resuscitation (CPR)
- Once the arrest team arrives there should be one team leader, usually the medical SHO or registrar; take orders only from him/her and from the anaesthetist
- When other doctors have arrived and are taking over or directing the CPR, you should try to insert a venous line (Venflon) and start a slow infusion of 5% glucose (*not* saline). You could then help with things like connecting up a

sucker for tracheal suction or taking a turn at cardiac massage or ventilation via the Ambu-bag.

> Once the CPR is established, inducing reversion to sinus rhythm and normal cardiac function is your next priority: if a defibrillator is available but you do not know the patient's rhythm it is reasonable to give a single DC shock of 200 joules. Continue with CPR as soon as the shock has been given and try to get an ECG rhythm recording as soon as possible. If the single, blind shock does not work, do not give any more shocks but continue with CPR until you have an ECG monitor connected; once you know what the rhythm is, follow the guidance on page 218 (Fig. 5.1).

Successful resuscitation

The patient should be moved as soon as possible to the CCU or intensive therapy unit (ITU) and should have a 12-lead ECG, CXR, blood gas analysis and blood sample for U&E.

Unsuccessful resuscitation

> **The decision as to how long to continue with resuscitation should be made by the medical SHO or registrar in charge of the arrest team. In general terms, it is not appropriate to continue prolonged resuscitation in a patient who shows no response to the team's efforts or who flickers rapidly from sinus rhythm to asystole/VF and back again. In such a case, 10 minutes' resuscitation is more than enough. Once the team leader has decided to abandon resuscitation he/she should announce this clearly, stop everyone's efforts and disconnect the ECG monitor.**

After resuscitation has been abandoned the house physician should check whether any relatives are present: if so they should be interviewed (preferably with a nurse present). When speaking to the nurses after an unsuccessful resuscitation, remember that they may have become friendly with the patient and the death might have upset them.

Other points

- If you have time, put on a pair of gloves at an early stage of the resuscitation procedure
- Be careful with needles and other sharps which often get tossed around at a cardiac arrest
- Remember that patients in nearby beds can hear what is going on: be careful what you say and how you say it

- After the procedure (successful or otherwise) a full, clear account of what went on must be written in the case notes: this must include the names of all doctors present and the names and doses of all drugs given
- When you are on call, you must be able to respond instantly to cardiac arrest calls. If you usually sleep in the nude, make sure you have some pyjamas or theatre clothing to hand which you can pull on quickly in the event of an arrest call.

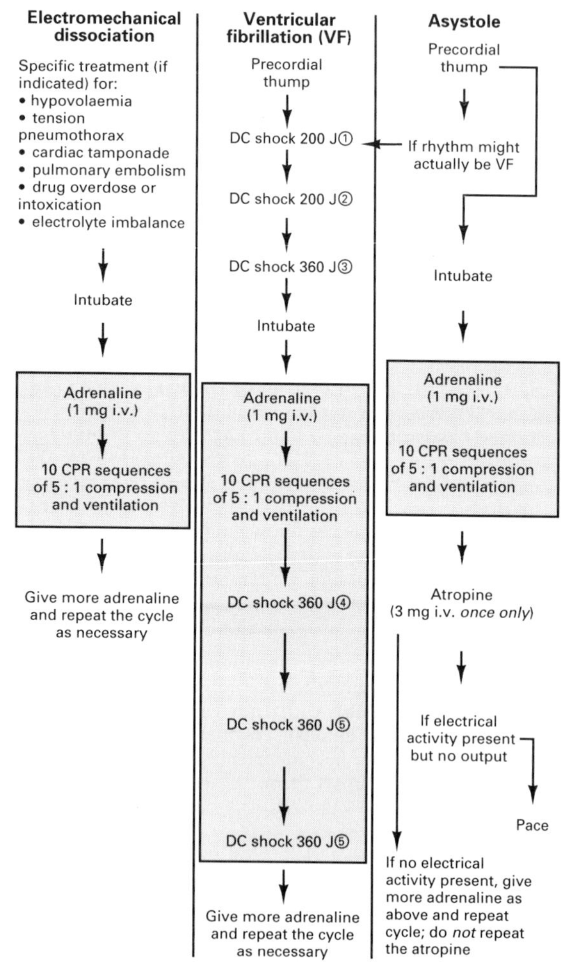

Fig. 5.1
Emergency resuscitation procedure.

MYOCARDIAL INFARCTION (MI)

Roughly half of all patients who die from an MI do so within the first 2 hours, so this condition must be treated with extreme urgency. The diagnosis of acute MI rests on the history.

DIAGNOSIS

The ECG may be *normal* in the early stages. In doubtful cases the ECG may give valuable supporting evidence (→ Figures 5.2, 5.3, 5.4, 5.5).

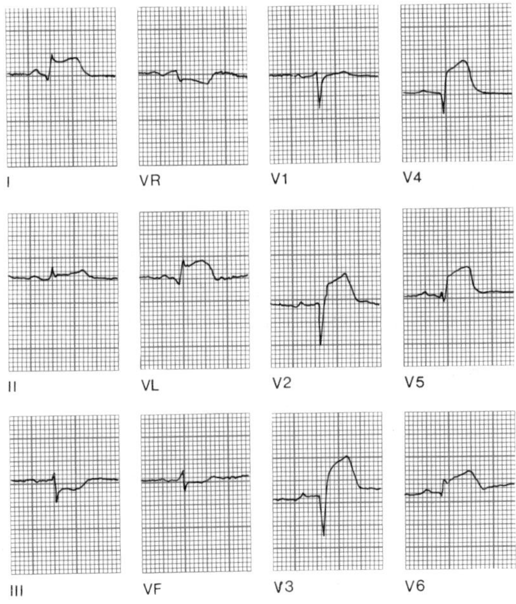

Fig. 5.2
Acute MI (anterior).

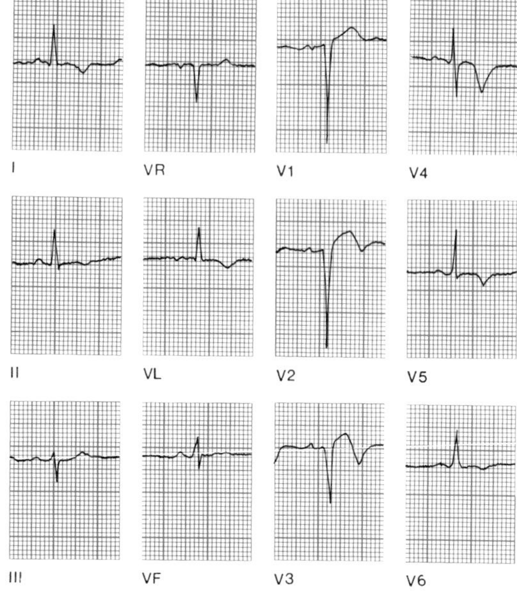

Fig. 5.3
Acute MI (anteroseptal).

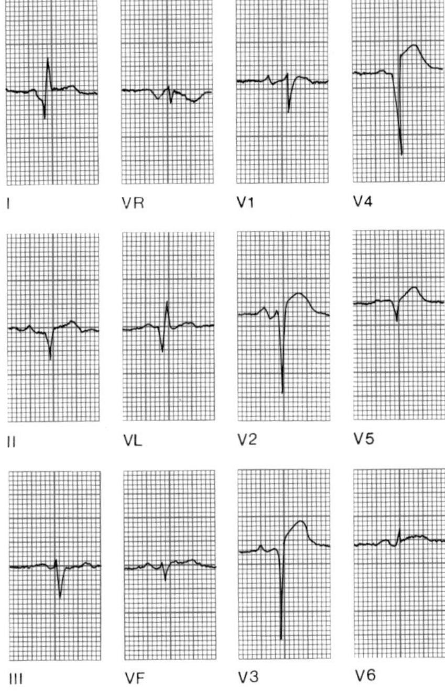

Fig. 5.4
Acute MI (anterolateral).

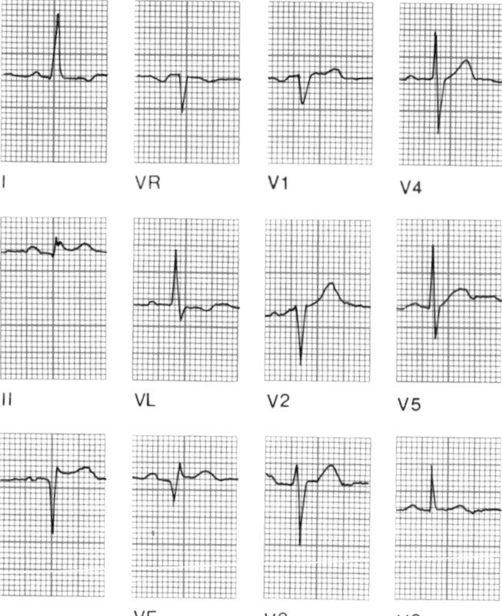

Fig. 5.5
Acute MI (inferior).

MANAGEMENT

Once you have decided that the patient has *definitely* or *probably* had an MI, the immediate priorities are:

1. Insert an intravenous cannula
2. Give analgesia in the form of diamorphine, 5 mg i.v. with prochlorperazine, 12.5 mg i.v. or metoclopramide, 10 mg i.v.
3. If a cardiac monitor is readily available (e.g. in the A & E department), connect the patient to it.
4. If there are no contra-indications (→Table 5.1), give streptokinase, 1.5 million units i.v. infusion over 60 minutes.

If pain subsides but then recurs, give further diamorphine. **If pain does not subside or recurs rapidly after diamorphine**, consider an intravenous nitrate infusion: provided the systolic BP is 100 mmHg or above, give intravenous isosorbide dinitrate, beginning at 2 mg per hour and increasing until pain is controlled. *Do not* continue increasing if systolic BP falls below 100 mm.

If the initial serum potassium is less than 4.0 mmol/l give an infusion of potassium chloride, 40 mmol diluted in 500 ml of 5% glucose over 4 hours. Use a programmable controller to ensure that the infusion does not run in too quickly.

If the patient develops ventricular ectopics these are likely to cause considerable anxiety to the nursing staff. Do not allow yourself to be persuaded to treat ectopics just because they are frequent or R-on-T in nature. The prognostic value of these features has been grossly exaggerated. If the ectopics are coming in salvos (which are, effectively, short runs of VT), treat with lignocaine: give a bolus of 100 mg i.v. over 2 minutes followed by an infusion (2 mg per ml in 5% glucose) at 4 mg per hour initially. Decisions about the further management of the infusion should be made in consultation with your SHO or registrar.

Table 5.1 **Contraindications to streptokinase**
Active peptic ulceration (bleeding within last 6 months)
Bleeding disorders (e.g. thrombocytopenia)
Recent surgery (within 10 days)
Invasive procedure (e.g. cardiac catheterization) within 10 days
Extensive cardiac massage
Proliferative diabetic retinopathy
Previous streptokinase within 12 months (use alteplase instead)
Systolic BP> 200 mm
Pregnancy (during the first 18 weeks)
Parturition (within 10 days)
Severe liver disease
Stroke (within 2 months)
Ulcerative colitis.
Menstruation
Infective endocarditis

ACUTE ASTHMA

Asthma can produce symptoms of all grades, from very mild to life-threatening; several hundred people die from asthma every year. It is, therefore, essential to treat it with respect and never to underestimate its dangers.

ASSESSMENT

History

You are probably dealing with a severe or potentially severe problem if:

- there is a history of several nights' sleeplessness resulting from shortness of breath
- the patient has had frequent hospital admissions for asthma
- the patient has been admitted to intensive care because of asthma
- the patient is on long-term oral steroids.

Examination

You should assess:

- the state of consciousness
- the patient's ability or inability to speak
- the degree of hyperinflation (visually), respiratory rate and pulse rate.

After the basic clinical assessment, ask the patient to record his/her peak flow measurement.

Potentially life-threatening features include:

- breathlessness so severe that the patient cannot complete a sentence in one breath or get up from a chair or bed
- respiratory rate of 25/min or more
- heart rate persistently above 110
- peak flow rate < 40% of predicted normal or of the patient's best result when well (200 litres per min if the patient's best is not known).

Imminently life-threatening features include:

- a silent chest on auscultation
- cyanosis
- bradycardia
- exhaustion, confusion or unconsciousness.

> ⚠ **It is possible to be severely hypoxic without being cyanosed.**

Investigations

- ABG (→ p 125) should be measured in all but the very mildest cases; remember to write on the request form the concentration of oxygen which the patient was breathing when the sample was taken.
- A CXR should be performed, chiefly so as to look for a pneumothorax, which is potentially a very serious complication of acute asthma.
- ECG in older patients (over 50) or those with a previous history of heart disease.
- Routine FBC.
- U & E (hypokalaemia is an important complication of treatment with beta-adrenergic agonists).
- Sputum for culture (if available).

MANAGEMENT

There is no place for therapeutic timidity in treating acute asthma: it is much better to treat very aggressively in the first 24–48 hours, then reduce the treatment later if appropriate.

Oxygen. High concentrations of oxygen (40% or more) should be given in all patients with pure asthma. In older patients who have chronic airways obstruction with some degree of reversibility (the area of overlap between asthma and chronic bronchitis), give 28% oxygen and repeat the blood gases 30 minutes later: if the PCO_2 is 6.0 kPa or less but the PO_2 is less than 10, increase the concentration of oxygen.

Inhaled beta-agonists. Give nebulized salbutamol, 2.5–5 mg or terbutaline, 5–10 mg. The nebulizer should be driven by oxygen unless there is concern about carbon dioxide retention, in which case air should be used. Repeat the nebulized beta-agonist every 4 hours.

Steroids. Give hydrocortisone, 200 mg i.v. at once followed by 200 mg i.v. every 6 hours. Once the patient can swallow, give oral prednisolone, 30 – 60 mg in the morning (there is no benefit in giving prednisolone in divided doses, except that the patient may have fewer tablets to swallow). After 24 hours from the start of the prednisolone you may stop the hydrocortisone.

Intravenous bronchodilators. If obviously life-threatening features are present give intravenous aminophylline, 250 mg over 30 minutes or a beta-agonist (salbutamol 200 μg or terbutaline 250 μg) over 10 minutes. A beta-agonist is preferred if the patient is already taking an oral theophylline.

Further management

In anyone with severe or very severe asthma a nurse or doctor should stay with the patient.

If the patient improves early on, continue with regular inhaled beta-agonist and with steroids as above.

If the patient has not improved after 15–30 minutes, give another dose of nebulized beta-agonist and add iprotropium bromide, 0.5 mg, to the nebulizer solution. *Contact your SHO or registrar.* A patient who fails to improve may need an intravenous infusion of aminophylline or salbutamol/terbutaline. Aminophylline infusion should be given by diluting 250 mg of the drug in 500 ml of 5% glucose and infusing at a rate of 0.5 – 0.9 mg per kg per hour (1 – 1.8 ml per kg/h). Thus, a 70-kg subject given 100 ml/h would be receiving about 0.7 mg/kg/h. If the patient's weight is not known, an approximate dose can be given according to Table 5.2:

Table 5.2
Approximate doses for varying weights

Small patients	600 – 100 mg per 24 h
Medium-sized patients	900 – 1500 mg per 24 h
Large patients	1100 –1900 mg per 24h

Salbutamol or terbutaline infusion should be given at an initial rate of 12.5 μg/minute (range 3 – 20 μg per min), adjusted according to peak flow rate and heart rate.

Severe hypokalaemia may occur during the treatment of asthma with high doses of beta-agonists. If you are giving thse drugs i.v., check serum K^+ every 6–12 hours.

Monitoring of progress

1. Repeat measurement of peak flow 15-30 minutes after starting treatment, then every 4 hours. Peak flow should be measured before each dose of nebulized salbutamol/terbutaline; some hospitals also measure peak flow soon after each dose of nebulizer, though in the opinion of the present author this is unnecessary and potentially confusing.
2. Repeat blood gas measurements within 2 hours of starting treatment, then 4-6 hours later if the patient's condition is not improving.
3. Keep a careful record of heart rate.
4. Measure the blood theophylline level if aminophylline is continued for more than 24 hours.
5. Measure serum K^+ (as above) and blood glucose.

Sedatives are absolutely contraindicated (except in an ITU) and antibiotics are not required in every case: they need only be given if the patient is febrile or has signs of focal infection in the chest. Percussive physiotherapy is contraindicated.

INDICATIONS FOR INTENSIVE CARE

- Hypoxia ($PO_2 < 8.0$ kPa) despite 60% oxygen or hypercapnia ($PCO_2 > 6.0$ kPa)
- Onset of exhaustion
- Confusion or drowsiness
- Unconsciousness
- Respiratory arrest
- Lack of adequate medical/nursing supervision on a general medical ward.

FOLLOW-UP CARE

Patients will not normally be discharged until their symptoms have cleared and breathing is virtually back to normal (peak flow > 75% of predicted or patient's best-known level). Treatment with inhaled steroids should be started at least 48 hours, and with bronchodilator inhalers 24–48 hours, before discharge. *Check that patients can use inhalers properly.* Talk to patients about how to tail off oral steroids and about measuring their peak flow rates at home. Some patients may require inhaled cromoglycate or an oral theophylline.

Reference. British Thoracic Society/Royal College of Physicians/King's Fund/ National Asthma Campaign. *British Medical Journal* 1990; 301 : 797- 800.

INFECTIOUS DISEASES

NOTIFICATION OF INFECTIOUS DISEASE

Doctors are required to notify the local consultant in Public Health Medicine of any patients who are suffering from certain infectious diseases: (→ Table 5.3)

Table 5.3
Infectious diseases requiring notification

Acute encephalitis	Ophthalmia neonatorum
Acute poliomyelitis	Paratyphoid fever
Anthrax	Plague
Cholera	Rabies
Diphtheria	Relapsing fever
Dysentery (amoebic or bacillary)	Rubella
Food poisoning	Scarlet fever
Leprosy	Tetanus
Leptospirosis	Tuberculosis
Malaria	Typhoid fever
Measles	Typhus
Meningitis	Viral haemorrhagic fever
Meningococcal septicaemia (without meningitis)	Viral hepatitis
Mumps	Whooping cough
	Yellow fever

If you know or strongly suspect that a patient has a notifiable disease you should ring the microbiology laboratory who will tell you the telephone number of the local Department of Public Health or Consultant in Communicable Disease Control (CCDC). If they cannot supply you with the number, try the hospital Infection Control Sister or the general administrative office. You should then fill in the appropriate form. In many cases, however, you will find that someone in your microbiology department has already 'notified' the patient.

Please note that AIDS (or the state of being HIV positive) is not a notifiable disease (→ also pp 23 – 25).

PROTECTIVE ISOLATION ('BARRIER NURSING')

Patients with certain highly infectious conditions, or who are suspected of having such a disease, are usually placed in single rooms and subjected to protective isolation or, as it is colloquially known, barrier nursing.

The list of diseases which require isolation is not the same as the list of notifiable diseases. Non-pulmonary tuberculosis, for example, is notifiable but does not require isolation.

Diseases which require the patient to be isolated are summarized in Table 5.4.

Table 5.4
Diseases requiring isolation

Brucellosis (with open lesion only)	Rubella
Chickenpox and shingles	Salmonella infection
Generalized herpes simplex	Shigella dysentery
Hepatitis A	Staphylococcal infections (highly resistant strains only)
Infectious diarrhoea (viral or bacterial)	*Streptococcus pyogenes* (heavy growth)
Measles	Tuberculosis (sputum smear positive only)
Meningococcal disease	Typhoid and paratyphoid fevers
Mumps	Viral haemorrhagic fever
Poliomyelitis	Viral meningitis
Pseudomembranous colitis	Whooping cough

It is worth remembering, however, that whilst isolation is an extremely valuable infection control measure, it is unpleasant for the patient and time-consuming for the nursing staff. Try, therefore, to discourage nurses from 'knee-jerk' isolation of any patient thought to have any kind of infection.

Patients needing isolation, will be accommodated in a single room. Anyone entering the room to touch or handle such patients or their urine, stools, vomit, etc. must put on a gown and gloves before entering the room. Having completed your work, you must discard the gown and gloves and wash your hands with an antiseptic *before* leaving the room. You should also make sure that the Infection Control Sister is made aware of the existence of these patients.

ANTIBIOTIC TREATMENT

The antibiotics used for the tratment of common infections are summarized in Table 5.5.

Table 5.5
Antibiotics for common infections

Disease	Drugs recommended
Septicaemia	
Unknown source	Gentamicin + metronidazole + ampicillin *or* cefuroxime (adjust according to possible primary focus of infection)
Neutropenia	Piperacillin + gentamicin (metronidazole should be added in cases of oral muscositis or perianal sepsis)
Meningitis	Benzylpenicillin or (if allergic) chloramphenicol
Gastrointestinal infection	
Diarrhoea	Nil (antibiotic rarely needed; consult microbiologist if in doubt)
Biliary tract infection	Cefuroxime
Peritonitis	Gentamicin + metronidazole + ampicillin *or* cefuroxime
Bone and joint infection	
Osteomyelitis, septic arthritis (not prosthetic joint)	Flucloxacillin + sodium fusidate
Respiratory tract infection	
Acute tonsillitis or pharyngitis	Penicillin V or erthromycin (many episodes are viral and do not need antibiotics)
Acute otitis media	Amoxycillin or erythromycin
Epiglottis	Chloramphenicol
Pneumonia — community acquired	Benzylpenicillin (+ erythromycin +/– rifampicin if severe) *or* erythromycin if 'atypical'
Pneumonia — aspiration	Cefuroxime + metronidazole
Exacerbation of COAD	Ampicillin or amoxycillin (a tetracycline or, in severe or non-responding cases, cefuroxime or co-amoxyclav)
Exacerbations of cystic fibrosis	Piperacillin + gentamicin
Skin and soft tissue infection	
Surgical wounds (lower GI or GU surgery)	Cephradine + metronidazole *or* ampicillin + flucloxacillin + metronidazole

Cellulitis	Benzylpenicillin + flucloxacillin (amoxycillin + flucloxacillin if oral) *or* erthromycin
Bites	Co-amoxyclav
Urinary tract infection	
Uncomplicated UTI	Trimethoprim *or* nitrofurantoin
Pyelonephritis	Gentamicin + ampicillin (*or* cefuroxime)
Prostatitis	Ciprofloxacin

Gentamicin nomogram

Instruction for use of the nomogram (Fig. 5.6):

1. Join with a straight line the serum creatinine concentration appropriate to the sex on scale A and the age on scale B. Mark the point at which the straight line cuts line C
2. Join with a straight line the mark on line C and the body weight on scale D. Mark the point at which this line cuts the dosage lines L and M.
3. The loading dose (mg) is written against line L. The maintenance dose (mg) and the appropriate time interval (hours) between doses are written against line M.

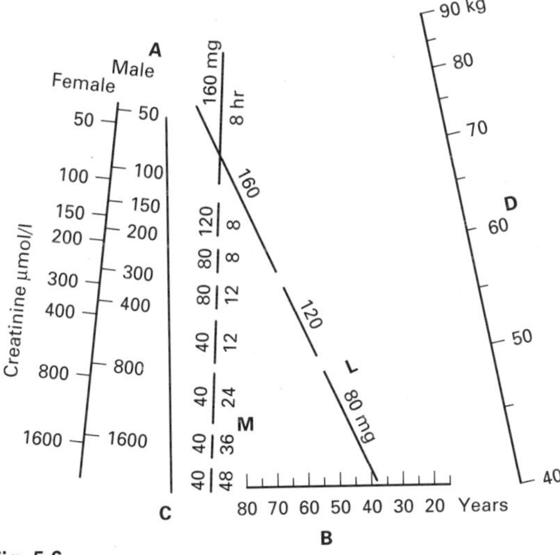

Fig. 5.6
The pre-dose level of gentamicin should not exceed 2 mcg/ml and levels 1 hour after the dose should be over 5 mcg/ml. Advice on dosage adjustment can be given by your local microbiologist. (Nomogram courtesy of Professor GE Mawer, University of Manchester.)

DIABETES

Diagnosis

Much mystery seems to surround the diagnosis of diabetes, but in fact this is straightforward in nearly all cases.

- Do not assume that someone has diabetes simply because you have found glycosuria. The diagnosis must be confirmed by a blood glucose measurement.
- Random blood glucose greater than 11 mmol/l or a fasting value greater than 8 mmol/l *and* symptoms of thirst and polyuria, mean the patient has diabetes by definition and there is no need to do a glucose tolerance test. Similarly, a random glucose less than 7 or a fasting value less than 6 excludes diabetes.
- Any patient with newly diagnosed diabetes who is in hospital should be referred to a specialist physician for assessment and follow-up. Errors are often made in judging the urgency of this referral: if the patient is well, has no ketonuria and has a blood glucose less than 20 mmol/l then the referral is not an emergency; on the other hand, if the patient is ill or has ketonuria (more than trace) then the situation is urgent irrespective of the level of the blood glucose. If a newly diagnosed diabetic has ketonuria then blood gases must be estimated urgently; if the plasma bicarbonate is less than 20 mmol/l the patient should be referred to the duty medical registrar as a case of ketoacidosis.

Monitoring of the diabetic state

The biggest single error that is made in monitoring is that blood glucose levels are not measured often enough: the blood glucose is much more variable in patients with diabetes (especially those treated with insulin) than in the non-diabetic population and it simply is not possible to guess the dose of insulin which the patient will require without adequate information. Reagent strips (BM glycemie stix, Glucostix, etc.) are perfectly adequate in most cases provided the tests are done by personnel who know how to use the sticks properly. Testing should normally be carried out before each main meal and before bed, though in acutely ill patients 2-hourly or even hourly testing may be necessary. In hospital in-patients testing the urine for glucose is *useless* as a means of monitoring diabetic control. The only reason for testing the urine is to look for ketones or, in some instances, for protein.

MANAGEMENT: NON-INSULIN-DEPENDENT DIABETES MELLITUS (NIDDM)

The primary treatment of NIDDM is diet, with the aim of reducing excess weight and avoiding refined sugar; tablets and insulin should not be used before an adequate trial of diet

(1 – 2 months) unless the patient is acutely ill or has a very high blood glucose (over 25 mmol/l), in which case you should consult a member of the hospital's diabetic staff or the duty medical registrar. In managing NIDDM it is important to look after the whole patient and not just to treat the blood glucose; in particular, the patient should be warned about the dangers of smoking and should receive vigorous treatment for hypertension or hypercholesterolaemia. The patient should also receive proper diabetes education, preferably from a trained diabetes specialist nurse.

Management: diabetes during intercurrent illness

If the illness is relatively mild (a minor stroke or heart attack, for example) it may be possible to continue the patient's normal treatment, but remember that, as a general rule, diabetes impairs healing and recovery from infection unless it is strictly controlled, i.e. one should be aiming for blood glucose levels below 9 mmol/l.

If the patient is moderately unwell but can still eat and drink it may be possible to manage simply by increasing the patient's doses of tablets or insulin; in the latter case the total daily dose should be increased by 10–20%, mainly by increasing the long-acting insulin. For example, if Mrs B is normally on Actrapid 8 units, Monotard 16 units in the morning and 6 of each in the evening, one would aim for something like Actrapid 8, Monotard 20 in the morning and, respectively, 6 and 8 in the evening. Again the aim should be to keep the blood glucose below 9 mmol/l. If there is any doubt that the patient can be adequately managed by minor adjustments to his/her normal treatment, it is safest to put him/her on four injections per day of insulin, viz a short-acting insulin before each meal and a long-acting (isophane or IZS lente-type) at bed-time: in this way adjustments to insulin doses are easily made if control is unsatisfactory.

Guidelines for four-injection therapy

If the patient has previously been on diet alone or diet plus tablets, one should start with 6 units of soluble insulin (Actrapid, Velosulin, Humulin S, etc.) before meals and 6 or 8 units of long-acting insulin (Insulatard, Monotard, Humulin I) at bedtime. If the patient is already on treatment with insulin, calculate the patient's total daily dose, increase it by 10–20% and divide this into four equal amounts. For example, in the case of Mrs B (above), who is normally on 8, 16/6, 6, the total daily dose is 36 units, so one could increase to 40 units given as 10 units four times daily.

If the patient is very unwell and cannot eat (but is not in ketoacidosis; see below) it is best to use a combined glucose/potassium/insulin infusion ('GKI regime'): to 500 ml of 10% glucose solution, add 2 g of potassium chloride solution and 16 units of soluble insulin, mix well and run in at 100 ml per hour using a programmable infusion pump. If the blood glucose level is not in the desired range (5–9 mmol/l) one should take down the bag and put up another one containing 20 units of insulin (for high blood glucose values) or 12 units of insulin (for low values). You should not attempt to correct the blood glucose by varying the rate of infusion of the cocktail: keep it at 100 ml per hour. If you are anxious to avoid fluid overload, use 20% glucose run at 50 ml per hour; if the patient is dehydrated, use 5% glucose at 200 ml per hour but in any event see that the insulin infusion rate is approximately 3 units/hour and that adequate potassium is supplied.

With a patient who has vomited and cannot eat at all the insulin must **NEVER** be stopped on the spurious grounds that lack of carbohydrate intake implies a lower insulin requirement. An ill diabetic requires more insulin than usual, not less. If you ignore this piece of advice the patient may die. Any insulin-dependent diabetic who is vomiting but in whom there is no obvious mechanical cause must be assumed to be in ketoacidosis.

Hypoglycaemia

Patients treated by diet alone cannot become hypoglycaemic as it is the treatment which leads to hypoglycaemia, not the disease.

Patients treated with sulphonylurea drugs (chlorpropamide, glibenclamide, tolbutamide, etc.) may experience hypoglycaemia which may be prolonged. Such patients may need not only a bolus dose of glucose (by mouth or intravenously) but also a glucose infusion which may need to be continued for several hours.

> If a patient is on insulin and is having frequent hypoglycaemic attacks you should ask yourself whether there is a pattern to the attacks: hypoglycaemia between 10 a.m. and lunch-time is due to too much short-acting insulin in the morning: reduce the dose by 2–4 units; hypoglycaemia between 2 p.m. and evening meal is due to too much long-acting insulin in the morning: reduce dose by 4–6 units; hypoglycaemia between the evening meal and midnight is due to too much short-acting insulin in the evening: reduce dose by 2–4 units; hypoglycaemia during the night or before breakfast is due to too much long-acting insulin in the evening: reduce dose by 2–6 units.

Diabetes and surgery

Diet- or diet/tablet-treated patients. For minor surgery no special precautions are required. It is prudent to check the blood glucose and electrolytes before surgery. Tablet-treated patients will have their tablets withheld on the day of operation and may be given small doses (4 or 6 units) of short-acting insulin subcutaneously if the blood glucose rises excessively postoperatively (i.e. above 15 mmol). The normal dose of tablets may be resumed once the patient is eating normally.

For major surgery it is important to admit the patient several days before operation for a full assessment, including CXR, ECG and U & E. Tablets should be stopped 24–48 hours pre-operation and the patient changed to four-times daily insulin, using 6 units of soluble insulin (Actrapid, Velosulin, Humulin S, etc.) before meals and 6 or 8 units of long-acting insulin (Insulatard, Monotard, Humulin I) at bed-time.

Wherever possible the patient should be first on the operating list. On the day of operation, take blood for glucose and U & E as early as possible, then set up a glucose/insulin/potassium infusion ('GKI regime'): to 500 ml of 10% glucose solution, add 2 g of potassium chloride solution and 16 units of soluble insulin, mix well and run in at 100 ml per hour using a programmable infusion pump. If the blood glucose level is not in the desired range (5–9 mmol/l) one should take down the bag and put up another one containing 20 units of insulin (for high blood glucose values) or 12 units of insulin (for low values). You should not attempt to correct the blood glucose by varying the rate of infusion of the cocktail: keep it at 100 ml per hour. If you are anxious to avoid fluid overload, use 20% glucose run at 50 ml per hour; if the patient is dehydrated, use 5% glucose at 200 ml per hour but in any event see that the insulin infusion rate is approximately 3 units/hour and that adequate potassium is supplied. Do not interrupt the infusion in order to give other fluids or blood. A GKI regime can be continued, if necessary, for a week or longer after operation and should be capable of maintaining good glycaemic control.

Once the patients are eating freely, they can be transferred back to four-times-daily insulin then back to tablets.

INSULIN-TREATED PATIENTS

For minor surgery the patient should receive the normal doses of insulin up to (and including) the evening before operation. On the morning of operation the patient should be given no soluble insulin but should receive about two-thirds of the normal dose of long-acting insulin together with an infusion of 10% glucose at 100 ml/hour.

For major surgery it is important to admit the patient several days before operation for a full assessment, including CXR, ECG and U & E. If the patient normally has a dose of insulin before the evening meal then on the day before operation the usual dose of short-acting insulin plus about two-thirds of the usual dose of intermediate- or long-acting insulin should be given.

Wherever possible the patient should be first on the operating list.

On the day of operation, take blood for glucose and U & E as early as possible, then set up a glucose/insulin/potassium infusion ('GKI regime'): to 500 ml of 10% glucose solution, add 2 g of potassium chloride solution and 16 units of soluble insulin, mix well and run in at 100 ml per hour using a programmable infusion pump. If the blood glucose level is not in the desired range (5–9 mmol/l) one should take down the bag and put up another one containing 20 units of insulin (for high blood glucose values) or 12 units of insulin (for low values). You should not attempt to correct the blood glucose by varying the rate of infusion of the cocktail: keep it at 100 ml per hour. If you are anxious to avoid fluid overload, use 20% glucose run at 50 ml per hour; if the patient is dehydrated, use 5% glucose at 200 ml per hour but in any event see that the insulin infusion rate is approximately 3 units/hour and that adequate potassium is supplied. Do not interrupt the infusion in order to give other fluids or blood. Do not use Hartmann's solution as it contains lactate. A GKI regime can be continued, if necessary, for a week or longer after operation and should be capable of maintaining good glycaemic control.

Once the patient is eating freely, institute four-times-daily insulin: take the patient's normal daily dose (in total), increase it by 10–20% and divide this total into four equal parts, giving a dose of short-acting insulin before each meal and a dose of long-acting insulin at bed-time.

When it is clear that the patient is recovering and is apyrexial, the normal insulin regime can be instituted.

Ketoacidosis and hyperosmolar, non-ketotic coma

These are both dangerous conditions with a significant mortality. In order to manage these emergencies properly you will need the help of a more senior colleague. The essential steps in management are:

1. Assess the patient's level of consciousness and vital signs (pulse, blood pressure and temperature).
2. Assess the patient's level of hydration but remember that most patients admitted in semi-coma or coma due to ketoacidosis are depleted of at least 6 or 8 litres of fluid.
3. Take blood for FBC, glucose, U & E, cultures and an arterial sample for gases.
4. Arrange an ECG and a CXR.
5. Try to find out from the patient or witnesses whether there are any clues as to the precipitating cause of the acute illness.
6. Give fluid in the form of normal (0.9%) saline. The first litre (without potassium) can be given as fast as it will run in; second and subsequent litres should have lots of added potassium (up to 20 mmol per hour) and can be given over 1–2 hours. Do not be misled by finding a normal serum potassium at presentation. The patient is almost bound to have a marked deficit in total body potassium.

7. If the serum sodium is greater than 150 mmol/l do not give normal saline but give fluid as half-normal (0.45%) saline.
8. Give insulin intravenously: a short-acting insulin (Actrapid, Velosulin, Humulin S) must be used. Begin with a bolus of 10–20 units (depending on the blood glucose) and follow this with an infusion of 6 units per hour, increased if necessary.

> The aim is to lower the blood glucose by about 10% per hour and to clear the acidosis. If the blood glucose has fallen to a low value (less than 11 mmol/l) but the patient is still acidotic (plasma bicarbonate less than 20 mmol/l), do not reduce the insulin infusion rate to very low levels; rather, keep it at 4 units/hour and give the patient 10% glucose by infusion (100 ml/h) instead of saline.

9. Very drowsy or unconscious patients should be admitted to a high-dependency unit and placed on a cardiac monitor.
10. Monitor the patient's condition by frequent (hourly or 2-hourly) measurements of blood glucose and U & E and urinary ketones.
11. Culture urine, sputum and any other available secretions, then start a broad-spectrum antibiotic.
12. Once the patient is clinically well, the urine is ketone-free and the plasma bicarbonate is > 20 mmol/l the insulin infusion rate may be reduced to 1–2 units per hour.
13. Do not attempt to change the patient from intravenous to subcutaneous insulin until the urine is ketone-free and the patient is able to eat normally; if the acidosis clears but the patient still does not feel like eating, use a GKI regime.
14. If the patient is in hyperosmolar, non-ketotic coma, hyperviscosity and thrombosis are major worries, so the patient should be anticoagulated with heparin unless there is a specific contraindication.

ALCOHOLISM

Patients who abuse alcohol may come your way because:

- They are admitted semi-comatose or comatose without any definite diagnosis.
- They take an excess of alcohol in addition to some other drug (e.g. paracetamol).
- They present to the A&E department with acute alcohol withdrawal (e.g. delirium tremens).
- They present with acute alcoholic hepatitis.
- They present with one or more epileptiform fits.
- They present with haematemesis due to peptic ulceration, alcoholic gastritis or oesophageal varices.
- They are admitted with another condition such as a chest infection, atrial fibrillation or unexplained heart failure and it becomes apparent within the first 24-48 hours that they have a problem with alcohol.

You should, therefore, have a high index of suspicion for alcohol abuse in any patient who presents with one of the above conditions. Alcohol abuse is especially common among men living alone, those with a history of depression and people in high-risk occupations such as publicans, commercial travellers, journalists and doctors.

HISTORY

1. Ask about the type of alcohol consumed and the amount: remember that one unit of alcohol is equivalent to half a pint of beer or lager, one single measure of spirits or a glass of wine. A standard 75 cl bottle of wine therefore contains 6 units of alcohol and a 75 cl bottle of spirits 30 units. The recommended weekly allowance of alcohol is 21 units or less for men and 14 units or less for women.
   If a patient appears very likely to be abusing alcohol but says to you: 'I used to drink a lot but I only have the occasional pint nowadays', the chances are that it is a lie.
2. Ask about the timing and circumstances of the drinking and try to fit this into a CAGE score (→ Table 5.6).

Table 5.6
CAGE Score

1. Have you ever thought you should CUT down on your drinking?
2. Have people ANNOYED you by criticizing your drinking?
3. Have you ever felt bad or GUILTY about your drinking?
4. Have you ever had a drink first thing in the morning (EYE-OPENER) to get rid of a hangover?

A CAGE score of two or more is said to identify the person as having a drink problem

Other useful questions include:

- Can you always control your drinking?
- Has alcohol ever led you to neglect your family or your work?
- What time of day do you start drinking?
- Describe a typical day's drinking.

EXAMINATION

Look out for:

- signs of chronic liver disease (spider naevi, clubbing, palmar erythema, Dupuytren's contracture, oedema, testicular atrophy)
- jaundice
- evidence of abnormal bruising
- evidence of cardiac arrhythmia, cardiomegaly or heart failure
- enlargement of the liver and spleen (hepatomegaly can occur in patients with cirrhosis, especially if there is a superimposed alcoholic hepatitis or fatty infiltration)
- a flapping tremor (coarse, low-frequency tremor of the hands when the arms are heldout in extension and the wrists dorsiflexed)
- evidence of mental clouding and disorientation. In addition to the usual questions about date, place, etc. it is useful to ask the patient to copy a five-pointed star; patients who have early hepatic encephalopathy may appear otherwise normal but fail badly on the five-pointed star test.

INVESTIGATIONS

In any patient with known or suspected alcohol abuse it is important to check an FBC, U & E, glucose, LFTs, clotting screen and (if there is a history of coma) CXR. If there is any history of abdominal pain you should also check a serum amylase. The sorts of abnormalities that you might expect to find are given below.

FBC. A high MCV, low platelet count (due to dietary folate deficiency), anaemia (due to a chronically poor diet).

U&E. Low sodium (during the acute phase of the illness), low urea. This latter is fairly specific for alcoholic liver disease, the only other common cause for a low urea being pregnancy.

Glucose. This may be low (< 3 mmol/l), *especially in the patient who has taken both alcohol and paracetamol.* The glucose may also fall abruptly, having been initially normal.

LFTs. There may be evidence of hepatitis, with a high bilirubin and raised transaminases. In early alcoholic liver disease the γGT is often raised even when the other liver enzymes are normal or nearly so. In later stages the serum albumin is usually low.

Clotting screen. The higher the PT and APTT (KCCT), the more severe is the liver disease

CXR. If the patient has been unconscious or has been lying on the floor for some time there may be segmental consolidation due to aspiration of vomit or due to infection. Long-standing alcohol abusers frequently develop infections due to unusual organisms, e.g. *Klebsiella*, and such people are at considerably increased risk of tuberculosis.

MANAGEMENT

Alcohol-related coma or semi-coma

1. Make sure that you have excluded other causes of coma (→ Table 5.7).

Table 5.7
Causes of coma

Most common	Stroke/TIA, sub-arachnoid haemorrhage, head injury, drug overdose (including alcohol), cardiogenic shock, cardiac arrhythmia, epilepsy
Common	Meningitis, poisoning (e.g. carbon monoxide), respiratory failure, renal failure, hepatic failure, shock 2° to blood loss, hypoglycaemia, hyperglycaemia (± ketoacidosis), encephalitis, hypothermia, subdural haematoma
Uncommon	Hypothyroidism, psychosis, hypercalcaemia

2. Nurse the patient in the 'recovery' (three-quarter prone) position.
3. If you suspect that the patient is a heavy alcohol abuser, has chronic liver disease or has taken paracetamol, ask the nurses to measure the blood sugar (capillary) every hour or 2 hours until stable.

Alcoholic hepatitis

Such patients often look unkempt, malnourished and covered in bruises; they are often febrile, even in the absence of obvious infection. They may be jaundiced and the liver is often acutely tender. Take blood for hepatitis A,B and C serology and, if the patient is febrile, for culture. Treatment is then supportive and consists of analgesia (*not* paracetamol or aspirin), fluids and observation.

Delirium tremens

This can be a very alarming condition, both for the patient and medical attendants. If severe it can progress to convulsions. If the patient is conscious and reasonably cooperative treatment should be by reassurance and by the use of chlordiazepoxide (Librium): the usual dosage schedule is given in Table 5.8.

Table 5.8
Chlordiazepoxide dosage

Days 1–2 ...... 15 mg 6 hourly
days 3–4 ...... 10 mg 6 hourly
days 5–6 ...... 5 mg 6 hourly
days 7–8 ...... 5 mg 8 hourly
days 9–10 .... 5 mg 12 hourly
days 11–12 .. 5 mg at night

You should also give large doses of thiamine, preferably by mouth (100 mg twice or three times daily). If clotting is abnormal, give vitamin K as menadiol, 10 mg orally once daily.

If the patient is malnourished or the history suggests chronic, severe alcohol abuse it may be necessary to give parenteral thiamine in the form of Parentrovite. This must be given *before* any i.v. glucose solution so as to avoid precipitating Wernicke's encephalopathy. Parentrovite has been known to cause severe anaphylactic reactions, albeit rarely, so it must be given by slow intravenous injection (over 10 min). Be sure to use the IVHP ampoules (not IMHP) if you are giving the drug i.v.

If the patient cannot swallow or is uncooperative it may be necessary to give chlormethiazole (Heminevrin) by infusion: using a standard 0.8% solution, give between 3 and 7.5 ml per minute until shallow sleep is induced, then reduce to 0.5 – 1 ml per minute to maintain shallow sleep.

Chlormethiazole infusion carries a significant risk of deep coma and respiratory depression. Patients treated in this way must be kept under close observation.

Fits

It is not necessary to administer anticonvulsants for a single fit; the patient can simply be treated with chlordiazepoxide and thiamine as above. If fits continue they should be treated by means of a chlormethiazole infusion.

Alcohol abuse discovered in the course of another illness

This is a remarkably common problem, especially in areas of high unemployment or social deprivation. The patient may need treatment with thiamine and chlordiazepoxide as above and, after recovery, should be offered counselling (→ below).

After the crisis

Any patient who has recovered from an acute episode of illness related to alcohol abuse is at high risk of relapsing if not offered support. Try to put the patient in touch with a local counselling service, the local branch of Alcoholics Anonymous or a psychiatrist with a special interest in the problem.

Reference. Mayfield D, McLeod G, Hall P. *American Journal of Psychiatry* 1974; 131:1121–1123.

OVERDOSES

Deliberate self-poisoning is a very common medical emergency. A few basic observations:

- Most people who take an overdose are not psychiatrically ill nor, contrary to popular opinion, are they uttering a 'cry for help' because of some overwhelming personal stress. The vast majority of such patients are immature, socially inadequate or have a personality disorder. Many overdoses are taken impulsively in response to relatively trivial stresses such as a row with a boyfriend.
- The truth of the above means that most doctors perceive overdose patients to be a bloody nuisance. However, mixed in with the dross will be a significant number of people who are psychiatrically ill or who have suffered a major personal stress. You must, therefore, treat each case on its merits.
- However much of a pain you find the average 'overdose' patient to be, a punitive or critical attitude does not do anything to reform the time wasters and is unfair and unhelpful to the patient who is in genuine distress. Try, therefore, to take a deep breath and keep your cool when going to see such patients.
- Patients who attempt suicide, often repeatedly, have a high rate of successful suicide whether they are psychiatrically ill or not. Repeated overdosage is, therefore, a bad prognostic sign and must be taken seriously.

In summary, therefore, you have a responsibility to assess the self-poisoned patient in two ways:

- in terms of drug toxicity
- in psychiatric terms.

BASIC APPROACH

If the patient is conscious and coherent ask:

- What has been taken?
- When was it taken?
- Was anything else taken apart from the main poison?
- What is the psychological and personal background (→ Table 5.9)?

Table 5.9
Psychological and personal backgrounds

1. Why did they do it?
2. Was the act premeditated or impulsive?
3. Did the patient intend to die?
4. Did the patient intend to be discovered?
5. Is there continuing suicidal intent?
6. Has the precipitating crisis resolved?
7. What are the patients' social circumstances and potential supports?
8. Are there any young children at home who might be at risk?
9. Can they identify anything which makes life worth living?
10. Have they harmed themselves before?
11. Is there a family history of suicide?
12. What are the main psychiatric symptoms (if any)?
13. Do they currently have a problem with alcohol or drug abuse?
14. Does the patient have a history of psychiatric disorder?
15. Are they expressing hopelessness?

INDICATIONS FOR PSYCHIATRIC REFERRAL

- Clinical depression present
- Psychosis (delusions/hallucinations/bizarre behaviour, etc.)
- Evidence of clear premeditation or continuing suicidal intent (the more detailed the plans the more serious the risk)
- Violent method chosen
- Alcoholics and drug addicts
- Older (over 45) and younger (under 16) age
- Serious or chronic physical illness present
- Those in a major life crisis which has not yet resolved
- Deliberate self harm (DSH) recidivists and those who have harmed themselves recently
- Any patient who gives you, the nurses or the family cause for concern.

If the patient is semi-conscious, unconscious or incoherent, before doing anything else you should:

- Make sure that you are not dealing with a cardiac arrest, i.e. check that the patient has a palpable carotid or femoral pulse.
- Note whether the patient is cyanosed or appears to have an abnormal breathing pattern (e.g. Cheyne-Stokes breathing). Check that the airway is clear.
- Check the BP.

If the patient's immediate survival seems in danger, call for help from your SHO or registrar.

If the patient's immediate survival is not threatened, try to obtain the answers to the above questions from a relative, friend or other witness.

EXAMINATION

Assess the patient's level of consciousness in terms of the GCS (→ p 102). Examine each system in turn, looking especially for:

- brady- or tachycardia
- BP
- abnormal respiratory pattern
- signs of peritonitis
- meningism
- papilloedema
- facial asymmetry or asymmetry of limb posture
- reflexes.

Patients who are unconscious or nearly so, should be nursed in the three-quarter prone position.

INVESTIGATIONS

- Take blood for salicylate and paracetamol levels in all patients (the history may be unreliable). If you know that the patient has taken paracetamol or a paracetamol-containing compound preparation (e.g. co-proxamol, Co-dydramol), do not take blood until after 4 hours from the time of ingestion.
- Take blood for U & E and blood glucose. This is especially important in paracetamol poisoning.
- In cases of paracetamol poisoning, take blood for a coagulation screen and for LFTs.
- In appropriate cases, take blood for levels of specific poisons, e.g. lithium, digoxin, theophylline, paraquat.
- In older patients (over 50) ask for an ECG.
- If the patient is unconscious ask for a CXR together with X-rays of any injured parts.

MANAGEMENT

General measures

1. If you are not familiar with the poison, consult the Data Sheet Compendium or the textbook on poisoning in the A & E department. If you are still unclear about its properties or if it is something peculiar (such as metal polish or a household chemical), contact your nearest Poisons Information Service (Table → 5.10).

Table 5.10
Poisons Information Services

London	071-635-9191 or 071-955-5095
Belfast	0232-240503
Birmingham	021-554-3801
Cardiff	0222-709901
Edinburgh	031-229-2477 or 031-228-2441
Leeds	0532-430715 or 0532-432799
Newcastle	091-232-5131

2. Gastric lavage: this is generally of value only if undertaken within 4 hours of ingestion. Lavage is worthwhile after long periods if certain drugs have been taken, however : up to 6 hours in the case of opiates and up to 12 hours for salicylates, tricyclic antidepressants and aminophylline. It must *not* be undertaken in those who have swallowed a corrosive or a petroleum product. If the patient is semi-conscious or unconscious the airway must be protected by means of an endotracheal tube (passed by an *experienced* person) before lavage is attempted.

Technique of gastric lavage. Carry out the following:

- have a suction apparatus ready to hand (check that it is working)
- lay the patient in the left lateral position
- raise the foot of the bed
- pass the lavage tube, asking the patient to swallow (get someone to show you how to do this before you make your first solo attempt)
- check that the tube is in place by blowing air down it and listening over the stomach
- wash out the gastric contents using 300 ml volumes of tepid water
- repeat until no more tablets are retrieved and the fluid is clear
- when pulling out the tube, pinch the distal end to prevent aspiration of fluid from the tube.

ANTIDOTES FOR SPECIFIC DRUGS

Paracetamol

This drug is freely available over the counter and is also present in many compound analgesics (co-proxamol, Co-dydramol, etc.). It is highly toxic in overdosage: deaths have resulted from the ingestion of as little as 10–15 gm (20–30 tablets).

Initial measures. Carry out the following:

- Take blood for U & E, glucose, clotting screen, paracetamol level and LFTs. (Note that the paracetamol level is only interpretable if it is measured 4 hours or more after ingestion).

- If the patient presents within 4 hours of ingestion, perform gastric lavage (→ above).
- If the patient refuses lavage or can swallow after the lavage, give 10 tablets (2.5 g) of methionine by mouth, followed by three further doses of 10 tablets every 4 hours.
- Check the patient's paracetamol level against the 'treatment line' on Figure 5.7.

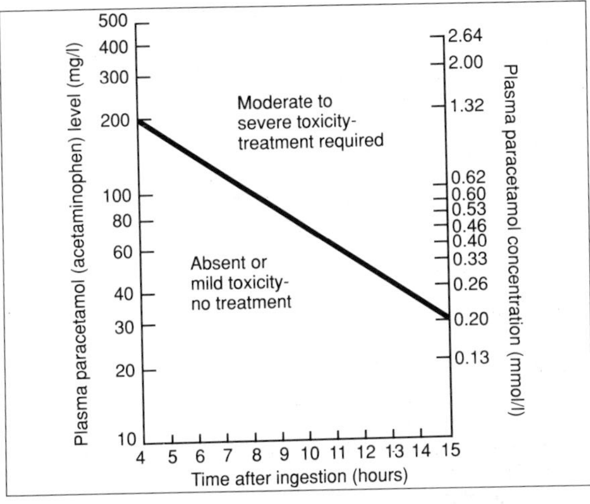

Fig. 5.7
Graph to indicate risk of hepatotoxicity from paracetamol poisoning as judged by plasma level.

If the level is *well below* the line, no specific antidote is required; if, however, the level is close to or above the line, give acetylcysteine (Parvolex) by i.v. infusion.

If the paracetamol level is doubtful, i.e. near the treatment line, it is safer to give acetylcysteine than not to give it.

Make up the acetylcysteine in 5% glucose (→ the package insert in the box) and give 150 mg/kg in 200 ml over 15 minutes, followed by 50 mg/kg in 500 ml over 4 hours, then 100 mg/kg in 1000 ml over 16 hours.

Do not begin acetylcysteine treatment if more than 15 hours have elapsed since ingestion.

Further measures. Carry out the following:

- Ask the nursing staff to measure blood glucose (capillary) every hour, then 4 hourly if stable.
- Check INR daily (more frequently in severe poisoning). The INR is the best overall guide to the extent of liver damage. If the INR exceeds 2.0 within the first 48 hours or exceeds 3.5 within the first 72 hours, ask for help from someone more senior.
- Review the patient carefully each day for signs of liver failure and check LFTs daily.
- Monitor urine output (catheterize if necessary) and check U & E daily.
- Do not discharge the patient less than 48 hours after admission because delayed liver damage is common. However, if the INR is normal at 48 hours, a well patient may go home.

Aspirin

This drug is freely available over the counter and is found in many compound analgesics. Symptoms of aspirin poisoning include tinnitus, hyperventilation, deafness, vasodilatation and sweating.

Aspirin poisoning dose not cause coma until a very late stage. Therefore severe poisoning can be present in a patient who is fully conscious.

Initial measures. Carry out the following:

- Take blood for U & E, acid/base state, clotting screen and salicylate level.
- Perform gastric lavage in all cases. Worthwhile recovery of tablets can result up to 24 hours after ingestion.
- If lavage is declined or after lavage has been performed, give activated charcoal, 5–10 g by mouth, repeated every 15–20 minutes until the dose of charcoal is 5–10 times that of the poison or until 50 g charcoal have been given.

Further measures. Carry out the following:

- If the plasma salicylate level is greater than 500 mg per litre (3.6 mmol/l), enhanced elimination is required. The traditional way to do this is by forced alkaline diuresis : give normal saline, 1 litre, with 40 mmol KC1, over 4 hours. Assuming that urine output is good (> 60 m/h) give:
  - 500 ml of 1.26% sodium bicarbonate, with 40 mmol KC1, over 4 hours
  - 500 ml of 5% glucose, with 40 mmol KC1, over 4 hours

– 500 ml of normal saline, with 40 mmol KC1, over 4 hours.
- Monitor urinary pH every 4 hours (try to keep it in the range 7.5 – 8.5) and plasma U & E every 4 hours.
- Repeat the cycle of fluids, 1 – 3, until two successive blood tests have shown a fall in salicylate level and the value is less than 300 mg/l (2.2 mmol/l).
  If there is any doubt about the patient's cardiac or renal function, forced alkaline diuresis should *not* be performed: haemodialysis should be considered instead
- Give vitamin K, 10 mg i.v., if the PT is prolonged.

Tricyclic antidepressants

The main dangers from these drugs when taken in overdosage are cardiac arrhythmias and conduction defects. Other effects include dry mouth, coma, hypotension, hypothermia, convulsions and respiratory failure. In severe poisoning there may be hallucinations, delirium and metabolic acidosis.

Initial measures. Carry out the following:
- Take blood for U & E, blood gases and acid/base state.
- Arrange a cardiac monitor.
- Give activated charcoal if the patient is conscious: 5–10 g by mouth, repeated every 15–20 minutes until the dose of charcoal is 5–10 times that of the poison or until 50 g charcoal have been given.

Further treatment. Carry out the following:
- Correct hypoxia.
- Correct acidosis (pH < 7.2) with intravenous 1.26% sodium bicarbonate, 500 ml initially.
- If the patient convulses, give i.v. diazemuls, 10-20 mg.
- Do not use antiarrhythmic drugs. Ask for help.

Benzodiazepines

This group includes diazepam (Valium), lorazepam (Ativan), nitrazepam (Mogadon), etc. They do not, as a rule, cause life-threatening effects unless the patient has chest disease or is in some other way at special risk from respiratory depression.

Management. Gastric lavage is not usually necessary. Treatment is essentially supportive; however, if you are concerned about respiratory depression, check arterial blood gases.

> If you think that a semi-conscious or unconscious patient may have taken an overdose of a benzodiazepine, a specific benzodiazepine antagonist (flumazenil [Anexate]) may be used as a diagnostic test : consult your SHO or registrar.

Iron

Poisoning is commonest in children and is usually accidental. Symptoms include : nausea; vomiting; diarrhoea; haematemesis; rectal bleeding. Hypotension, coma and hepatic necrosis may occur later.

Initial management. Carry out the following:

- Empty the stomach as quickly as possible, preferably by inducing vomiting.
- Perform gastric lavage and leave in the stomach a solution containing 5-10 g of desferrioxamine in 50-100 ml water.
- Take blood for serum iron measurement.

Further measures. Give desferrioxamine by intravenous infusion at a rate of 15 mg/kg/hour (maximum 80 mg/kg in 24 hours).

Opiates

These drugs cause coma and respiratory depression. Overdosage can be recognized by the presence of pin-point pupils.

Management. Carry out the following:

- Carefully assess pulse, BP rate and depth of respiration.
- Give naloxone, 0.8–2 mg i.v. as a bolus.
- If ventilation appears inadequate, check ABG.
- Make sure that the patient is going to be closely supervised by a nurse or doctor.
- Repeat naloxone every 2–3 minutes until breathing is adequate (up to a maximum dose of 10 mg). Alternatively, naloxone can be given by continuous i.v. infusion: dilute 2 mg in 500 ml of 5% glucose and give at a rate of 25 ml/minute, adjusted according to response.

Naloxone may precipitate symptoms of opiate withdrawal in addicts, e.g. tremor, sweating, abdominal pain, hallucinations: sedation with thioridazine may be required. High-dose opiate misusers may require methadone to combat withdrawal.

Overdosage of co-proxamol (Distalgesic): this drug contains an opiate (dextropropoxyphene) combined with paracetamol. It is very dangerous if taken in overdose. The initial features are those of opiate toxicity with coma, respiratory depression and pinpoint pupils; in severe cases cardiovascular collapse may occur. Early use of naloxone is essential. Paracetamol toxicity may occur later and acetylcysteine should be used when appropriate (→ above).

Phenothiazines

These drugs cause less depression of consciousness than other sedative drugs. Hypotension, hypothermia, sinus tachycardia and arrhythmias may occur. Dystonic reactions (rigidity, oculogyric crises, etc.) may occur even with quite small doses. In severe poisoning convulsions may occur, as phenothiazines lower the fit threshold.

Management. This is largely supportive, paying special attention to respiration, airway and BP. Patients should be connected to a cardiac monitor if they are:

- over 40
- have taken a large overdose:
- have any history of heart disease.

Severe dystonic reactions can be treated with procyclidine, 5–10 mg i.m., repeated if necessary after 20 minutes, or 5 mg i.v.; it is usually effective within 5 minutes. Alternatively, give benztropine, 1–2 mg i.m. or i.v., repeated if symptoms reappear.

Adverse reaction. Neuroleptic malignant syndrome is not a consequence of overdosage of phenothiazines as such but is a rare, very serious idiosyncratic reaction to neuroleptic drugs, including haloperidol, chlorpromazine and flupenthixol (Depixol). It consists of hyperthermia, fluctuating consciousness, muscular rigidity and altered autonomic function with pallor, tachycardia, labile BP, sweating and urinary incontinence. It is potentially fatal so if you think that a patient has the syndrome consult your SHO or registrar immediately.

Paraquat

Concentrated liquid paraquat (Gramoxone) is used by farmers and commercial gardeners. It is extremely toxic. The granular form (Weedol), used by amateur gardeners, contains only 2.5% paraquat and is less dangerous.

Ingestion of liquid paraquat is followed by nausea, vomiting and diarrhoea, then by painful ulceration of the tongue, lips and throat. Renal failure may ensue at this stage.

Management. Treatment should be begun immediately, with oral administration of Fuller's earth or bentonite to absorb the drug and reduce absorption. The stomach is then emptied by careful lavage and you should leave in the stomach 300 ml of a suspension containing 30 g of Fuller's earth and 15 g of magnesium sulphate. Take blood for U & E and FBC and contact your SHO or registrar immediately.

Amphetamines

These cause wakefulness, excessive activity, paranoia, hallucinations and hypertension, followed by exhaustion, hyperthermia, convulsions and coma. In the early stages chlorpromazine and beta-blockers may be useful. At a later stage tepid sponging, anticonvulsants and artificial ventilation may be necessary.

Index

A

B

C

D

E

F

G

H

I

J

K

L

M

N

O

P

Q

R

S

T

U

V

W

X

Y

Z

USEFUL TELEPHONE AND BLEEP NUMBERS

Consultant ______________________

Consultant ______________________

Consultant ______________________

Consultant ______________________

Consultant ______________________

Consultant ______________________

Senior Registrar ______________________

Registrar ______________________

SHO ______________________

Anaesthetist ______________________

Accident & Emergency ______________________

Administrator ______________________

Biochemistry ______________________

Blood Transfusion Service ______________________

Cardiology ______________________

Chest Physician ______________________

Cytology ______________________

Dentist ______________________

Dermatology ______________________

ENT ______________________

Gastroenterology ______________________

Haematology ______________________

Immunology ______________________

Microbiology ______________________

Neurology ______________________

Nursing Officer ______________________

Paediatrics ______________________

Pathology ______________________

Pharmacy ______________________

Porters ______________________

Renal medicine ______________________

Social Worker ______________________

Virology ______________________